D0774165

THE FEEL GOOD FACTORY ON

healthy living

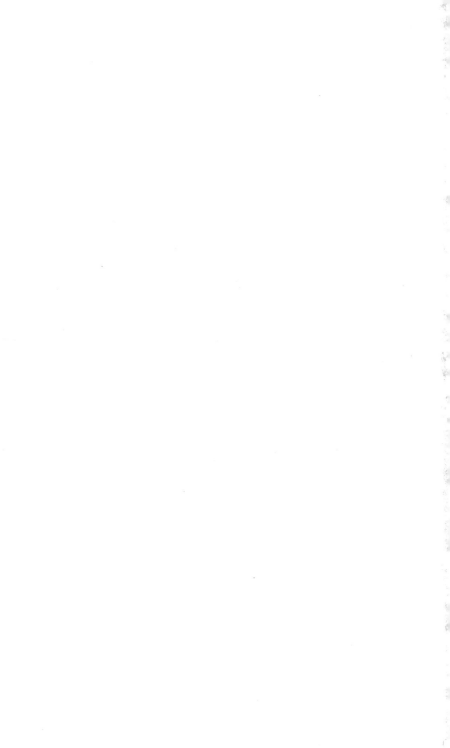

THE FEEL GOOD FACTORY ON
healthy living

Feel Good Factory led by Elisabeth Wilson

MANUFACTURED BY
THE FEEL GOOD FACTORY

First published in 2009 by
Infinite Ideas Limited
36 St Giles
Oxford
OX1 3LD
United Kingdom
www.infideas.com

A CIP catalogue record for this book is available from the British Library

ISBN 978-1-906821-22-7

The publisher would like to thank Kate Cook, Sally Brown, Jackee Holder and
Elisabeth Wilson for their contributions to this book.

Designed by D.R.Ink
Typeset by Sparks, Oxford – www.sparkspublishing.com
Printed and bound in Malta

Contents

Two: Making the changes

Three: Healthy and energised

Four: Optimum health

Introduction

This book works on the principle that making very small changes will reap huge health benefits. For a taste of how easy it is, put into action the ideas here.

We can't live for ever but we can live for a whole lot longer than our grandmothers would ever have believed possible. A baby girl born in the last decade, if she can reach the age of 60 without cancer or heart disease, can expect to live into her mid-90s. And that all-important bit, getting to 60 without major disease, has also never been more feasible. Because we now know that although genes play a part in our risk of succumbing to disease, a whopping 70–80% of that risk is down to factors over which we have control.

Isn't that empowering? Your life really is in your hands. By making decisions about how you live your life you can add years and years to it. And not just any old dismal years but happy, healthy, youthful years.

The main principle behind this book is straightforward: by making small decisions on a daily basis you can become healthier. This book is full of ideas for what these decisions should be. Adopt just a few of them and you'll look and feel better fast. Take on a new one each day for the next month and you'll transform your health – and ultimately your life – now and for years to come.

Follow the advice here and you will be hitting all the targets set by experts for exercise, nutrition and rest. These are the foundations on which good health is built. When you're in your 20s you can survive and thrive on a rubbish diet, no exercise and no sleep, but by the time you are in your 30s, the cracks will begin to show. We need to sort these three elements out if we want to enjoy any sort of quality of life; otherwise we'll run the risk of succumbing to the twenty-first century lifestyle illnesses: stress, exhaustion, depression. And more to the point, we'll be draining away time and quality from our later years. The decisions you make today will be impacting your life in years to come.

The focus of this book is on doing what you need to in order to feel energised, relaxed, calm and in control – and you can achieve that very quickly. The results are cumulative. Exercise – even a very little exercise – will help you sleep better. Once you're not so exhausted, you'll find the energy to eat better. When these three are in place in a rudimentary way, you can pick up on some of the fine tuning: popping a supplement; giving some attention to your emotional health; beating bloat for good.

There are lots of clever little tricks here that you can start on right away. One last thought: if you don't look after your health now, today, imagine what you'll look and feel like in 5 years, 10 years, 20 years time? Nothing is more important than you taking the time to look after yourself. Start today. It's easy.

One

The basics

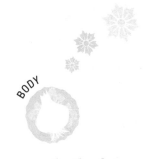

BODY

Be healthier by tomorrow

Motivated by instant results? These simple lifestyle changes, implemented throughout the day, could add years to your life.

There are many different ways to get healthier, live longer and look younger – by eating different foods, cutting others out of your diet, exercising, getting out and about, watching your stress levels and taking the right vitamins. You'll find simple ideas for tackling all of these within these pages.

But if you just want to get on with it, or you'd like to see what a healthier day might look and feel like, plunge right in with this programme. You'll soon see it's not too scary.

7.30 a.m. Always start your day with breakfast. People who eat breakfast live longer than people who don't – as long as they choose wholegrain-based cereals. Add a cup of green tea and a piece of fruit to boost your levels of disease-fighting antioxidants.

7.45 a.m. Drink a glass of water and take a multivitamin. Most people don't get the recommended daily allowance of many essential vitamins and minerals. You're more likely to remember to take a supplement every day if you take it with breakfast.

8.00 a.m. Brush and floss your teeth. It can take six years off your biological age. The bacteria that cause gum disease also cause furring of the arteries which can lead to heart disease.

8.30 a.m. Walk to work. Exercising for at least 30 minutes every day is the best way to keep your heart and lungs in good shape (not to mention the rest of you).

People who eat breakfast live longer than people who don't

9.00 a.m. Drink a glass of water and try to have six more throughout the day.

10.00 a.m. Have another cup of tea. Always squeeze your teabag – you'll release twice as many antioxidants.

10.30 a.m. Connect with your friends and colleagues by email or phone. People with a strong social network of friends and family live longer and healthier lives than more solitary types.

12.30 p.m. Do some lunchtime yoga. It balances out all the body's systems and gets your organs working efficiently. Ever wondered why yoga teachers look so young?

1.30 p.m. Have a rainbow salad for lunch. Use as many differently coloured vegetables – red peppers, watercress, grated carrot, courgette, spinach leaves, cherry tomatoes – as you can. Dress with olive oil and balsamic vinegar, and sprinkle with a handful of toasted sunflower and sesame seeds for the perfect antioxidant-packed, disease-fighting lunch.

3.30 p.m. Take the stairs. Climb up and down a flight six times a day and you'll prevent weight gain of 2kg a year. You take 36 days off your life for every 5kg overweight you are.

6.00 p.m. Meditate on the train home. You'll lower your blood pressure and slow your heartbeat, both of which are good for your heart's health. Close your eyes and breathe deeply, in through your nose and out through your mouth. Try to empty your mind and simply concentrate on what the breath feels like as it enters your nostrils and leave through your lips. Feel it filling your lungs and pushing out your abdomen. Keep this focus for around 10–15 minutes.

7.00 p.m. Have a small glass of red wine. Go for a deep red like a Pinot Noir for a maximum boost of disease-fighting flavonoids. Just be sure to stop at one or two.

8.00 p.m. Have salmon for dinner. Oily fish like salmon, or mackerel, sardines, trout or tuna, keep your brain healthy and can stave off Alzheimer's if eaten at least twice a week.

9.00 p.m. Watch a funny DVD. Laughter boosts your immune system and reduces the ageing effect of stress hormones on the body.

10.00 p.m. Have sex. People who have sex more than twice a week live longer than those who don't.

11.00 p.m. Sleep. It's your body's chance to release growth hormones and repair itself from the inside out. So never skimp on your shut-eye – aim for at least six to eight hours a night.

BODY

Start exercising when you really don't want to

Exercise keeps you calm, keeps you energetic, keeps you young and more than anything else will keep you long-term healthy. Here is how to get started and stay started.

Research shows that when life gets busy, exercise is one of the first things to get bumped off the schedule. But before you berate yourself for your lack of sticking power, it's good to remember that, even for professionally fit people like personal trainers, exercise is cyclical. There will be times when it gets pushed to the sidelines. However, for those who have learned how much exercise helps them cope with a busy life, the gaps before they start exercising again are likely to be shorter. If you've never exercised regularly, this idea aims to get you to a stage where you too can appreciate the benefits – and it isn't worth going without it for too long. It's great if you are a lapsed exerciser – it is so easy that you will mentally get back into the frame of mind without much effort, and your muscles won't have forgotten. You will get back to being fit quickly.

According to research, there are two reasons that exercise programmes fail:

- We don't see the results we want; or
- We set our expectations too high.

It's far better to do a little and stick to it until you have the exercise habit than go nuts, join a gym, write an ambitious exercise programme and then give up completely after a couple of weeks of failing to keep to it.

Decide on your goal

If you've never exercised consistently before, or haven't for a long time, start with a modest goal. If it's 10 minutes of activity a day – that's brilliant, as long as you are confident you will do it. Aim to visit your local pool once a week and get into the habit of doing that before you aim for three times a week. Or aim to swim once a week, and walk round the park once a week. It's better to make one yoga class on a Saturday morning rather than kid yourself that you'll make the 6 a.m. class three mornings a week before work.

You have to have a plan

You need a schedule where every week you are aiming to do a little more, a little more frequently until you are exercising for around three to four hours a week, enough to get you out of breath for most of the time. That could take a year, but don't think about that now. Stick your monthly schedule on the fridge. At first your goal should be just to stick to your weekly plan. Once you've got the hang of it, you can make your goal bigger such as: run around the park, undertake your local fun run, cycle to the next town then cycle back.

If you are very exhausted, very unfit, have been ill or are very overweight, all you might be able to manage is walking up a couple of flights of stairs. Fine. Make that your goal: to walk up stairs three times a week, then five times a week, and so on from there. Aim for cardiovascular exercise to begin with that gets your heart beating, because that's the type that will give you energy faster and help you to continue.

It's far better to do a little and stick to it

Here is a programme for a walker. Adapt it for whatever exercise you prefer.

- Week 1. Walk slowly for 5 minutes, walk briskly for 5 minutes, walk slowly for 5 minutes. Aim to do that 3 times a week.
- Week 2. Aim to do the same 5 times a week.
- Week 3. Walk slowly for 10 minutes, walk briskly for 10 minutes, walk slowly for 10 minutes. Aim for 4 times a week.
- Week 4. Walk slowly for 5 minutes, walk briskly for 20 minutes, walk slowly for 5 minutes. Aim for 5 times a week.

This may seem ridiculously easy but the point is to get back into the habit, not train for a marathon. Once exercise is part of your life, you can walk faster, walk further, start running for blocks of time, until you are finally reaching the level of exercising at a moderate level for 30 minutes most days of the week. Of course, you don't have to stick to walking/running, you can mix and match with other enjoyable forms of activity – a knock about with the kids counts if you move quickly and long enough.

Think FIT

Remember the acronym FIT: Frequency, Intensity, Time. When drawing up your plan, start working on frequency – aim to some form of exercise five or six times a week. Then work on 'T' – the time you spend at it each time you do it. Then move onto intensity – use hills to make you work harder or go faster, or try a more difficult stroke if you're swimming.

What about weight loss?

Of course, one of the primary reasons we exercise is to lose weight. Hint: when you are starting off, put ideas of losing weight out of your head. Studies show that those who exercise with the goal of losing weigh are far more likely to give up. It's that thing about expectations again. You have to exercise really pretty hard for weight loss; about six hours of running at a moderate pace every week. Concentrate instead on how much better you'll feel about yourself and how much energy you'll have. You begin to feel better within days of starting an exercise programme. It is this fantastic boost to mood and sense of self-esteem that helps people lose weight when they first begin exercising because naturally they steer towards nutritious food: the exercise habit underpins their intentions to lose weight. Of course, as you become a regular exerciser your metabolism will be boosted and the exercise will help you lose weight and, more important, maintain your new ideal.

Buddy up

And if all else fails, find a friend to exercise with. Research shows that those who make exercise dates with a friend are far more likely to stick to their programme and achieve their goals.

Quiz:
Are you younger than you think?

How fast you age is a process that's under your control far more than was thought before. How long your body and mind stay fit, active and healthy is determined by the choices you make. It's thought that you can have a biological age of 50 in your 70s.

Start with your chronological age and add or subtract.

Do you get at least 30 minutes of moderate exercise (such as walking) on most days?

Yes – subtract 1 year

Do you exercise intensively on a regular basis?

Yes – add 3 years

Do you rarely, if ever, do any physical exercise?

Yes – add 2 years

Are you more than 10% over the recommended weight for your height?

Yes – add 3 years

Are you the correct weight for your height?

Yes – subtract 1 year

Are you under stress or pressure on a regular basis?

Yes – add 4 years

Do you actively practise stress-reducing techniques such as meditation or yoga?

Yes – subtract 3 years

Have you experiences three or more stressful life events in the past year (for example, divorce, bereavement, job loss, moving house)?

Yes – add 3 years

Do you smoke?

Yes – add 6 years

Do you have a cholesterol level of 6.7 or higher (or has your doctor told you that you should think of reducing your cholesterol levels)?

Yes – add 2 years

Do you have blood pressure that's 135/95 (or has your doctor told you that you should think of reducing your blood pressure)?

Yes – add 3 years

Do you eat five or more portions of a range of fresh fruit and vegetables every day?

Yes – subtract 5 years

Do you regularly eat processed packaged or fast food?

Yes – add 4 years

Are you a vegetarian?

Yes – subtract 2 years

Do you eat oily fish three times a week?

Yes – subtract 2 years

Do you drink two or three small glass of red wine up to five days a week?

Yes – subtract 3 years

Do you drink more than 14 units of alcohol a week?

Yes – add 5 years

Do you have an active social life and supportive network of friends and family?

Yes – subtract 2 year

Do you have an active sex life?

Yes – subtract 2 years

Are you happily married?

Yes – subtract 1.5 years

If you're younger than your chronological age, keep up the good work, but if you're older, don't panic. There is a great deal you can do to strip years from your body and make it resistant to disease. Read on.

BODY

Drinking your way healthy

Dehydration is a major cause of lack of energy and minor health problems. Sort it out with this simple plan.

Only a lamentable one in ten of us are drinking the 1.5 litres a day of fluid that we should be (and when it's hot, when we exercise and we're ill, that should be 2 litres). Are you drinking enough? Water is the best hydrator of all, mainly because it's got nothing in it that needs to be processed by your body so it supplies the fluid without any stress on your hard-working organs. The simplest way of ensuring that you're drinking enough is to check your urine from mid-morning onwards: it should be straw-coloured.

If you don't drink enough, you get very tired. You may also overeat, as we often mistake thirst for hunger. Try drinking a cup of water ever hour and you might find your appetite for snacks decreases. You should also find that your need for tea and coffee reduces automatically.

Which brings us to caffeine. Tea and coffee have the benefit of supplying caffeine, which make us more alert. Except it doesn't. A recent study has discovered that caffeine doesn't actually work to make us more alert if we drink it regularly. It only has an effect on occasional users. What isn't in dispute (yet) is the effect that caffeine can have on physical performance. Sip an espresso or energy drink half an hour before exercising and you're likely to push harder and achieve more.

Coffee and tea are no longer the 'bogeys' they were once thought to be when it comes to hydration. For years we've heard that they are diuretic, causing us to lose fluid. But now that advice has been changed. The water in tea and coffee actually does contribute to hydration unless you really overdo it. In summary: the story on caffeine changes every month, but drinking around four cups of ordinary strength coffee or six cups of ordinary strength tea, doesn't appear to do any harm and may do some good.

If you don't drink enough, you get very tired

Instead of seeing getting enough good quality fluid as a chore, see it as an opportunity. Each glass or cup is its own little ritual, giving your well-being and energy levels a fillip. Stop. Sip. Savour.

7 a.m. Glass of hot water with the juice of a quarter of a lemon squeezed into it (a naturopath pick-me-up for your digestion and liver).

8 a.m. Glass of water to wash down your multivitamin and daily fish oil supplement taken after breakfast.

11 a.m. A cup of rooibos tea. This South African tea is loaded with antioxidants, and its distinctive taste makes it a great substitute for coffee addicts.

1 p.m. Cup of green tea after lunch. It helps rev up your metabolism, and those who drink four cups a day are less likely to suffer from brain ageing.

3 p.m. Glass of water with an effervescent vitamin C tablet – vitamin C wakes you up.

5 p.m. A glass of sparkling mineral water cut with fruit juice. Think of it as a cocktail to start your sparkling evening.

7 p.m. A cup of mint tea after dinner – try crushing your own mint leaves in a glass of hot water or bung in a teabag. Great for your digestion.

9 p.m. A cup of chamomile tea to soothe you off to sleep.

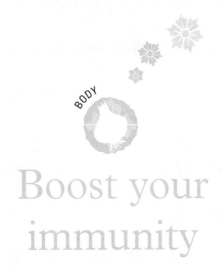

BODY

Boost your immunity

What exactly is your immune system, and how can you help it?

Your body has developed a highly effective defence system for keeping you healthy. Inside the body is an army of scavenging white blood cells, constantly roaming the corporeal highways and byways looking for invaders. If a scavenging cell spots an intruder, then it's immediately transported to the nearest lymph gland (situated in the neck, armpits and groin) and destroyed before it's even had a chance to wave a white flag. (You can feel this brutal elimination process taking place when your lymph glands become swollen.)

A healthy body with a fully functioning immune system sees off potentially dangerous organisms and carcinogens every day. It's even thought that cancer cells grow and are destroyed by the immune system on a regular basis. It's no surprise that a recent study of healthy centenarians found they had one thing in common: a healthy immune system.

The danger for most of us comes when the immune system is weakened and invaders remain undetected and start to multiply. But in most cases there are three main factors which lead to weak links in your inner defences: a less than ideal diet; the environment in which you live (constantly challenging your defences over and above what's normal by smoking, sunbathing or breathing polluted air); and mental well-being – feeling under stress on a regular basis.

You are what you eat

Your immune system works best when you keep it supplied with a full range of micronutrients such as vitamins and minerals. But even people who eat a balanced diet often show deficiencies and there are two theories as to the cause. When we evolved we were designed to lead active lives, hunting, gathering and escaping predators, and consuming 3000–4000 calories a day. Now we're mainly sedentary, and need around 2000 calories, we may not be eating enough to get the full range of micronutrients we need. The second theory is that today's intensive farming methods have depleted our soil of key minerals such as selenium and food processing methods further deplete food of micronutrients. We now know that a large number of people are regularly missing out on vitamins A, D and B12; folic acid, riboflavin, iron, magnesium, zinc, copper and omega-3 oils. Additionally, nutritionists think we're more likely to have deficiencies as we get older, because the digestive system become less efficient at absorbing micronutrients from the food we eat. So what we can do?

Take a supplement

Strengthening your immune system starts with taking a good multivitamin and mineral supplement every day. Supplements are one of those daily tasks that fall by the wayside. One quick tip is to keep supplements on your

Feel good now: *Stock up on flaxseed oil. It activates the hormone leptin, which is thought to speed up the metabolism. Drizzle the oil on porridge, salad or vegetables, or swallow a couple of spoonfuls neat. Healthy oils curb cravings, too.*

bedside table rather than the kitchen drawer. It seems that you remember to take them then and you need to top up your micronutrients ever day for benefits. This really helps: there was a US study that discovered that in people with weakened immune systems, taking a daily nutritional supplement achieved a fully functioning immune system within a year.

Be aware of your environment

Your body has a regular army designed to fight off everyday invaders, and it also has a troop of 'special forces' called T-cells, held in reserve for extraordinary circumstances. But if you bombard your body with extra invaders on a regular basis, the effectiveness of these special forces is inevitably weakened, allowing disease-causing bugs to multiply. And while you can't control the many bacteria and viruses that assault your immune system every day, you do have control over additional toxic invaders such as cigarette smoke (whether first-hand or passive) and, to a lesser extent, environmental pollution.

Have a massage

If you are feeling stressed on a regular basis it is as if you are offering a personal invitation to foreign invaders to walk through the chinks it causes in your defences. Many of the hormones involved in your body's fight or flight response – how it responds to stress – are actually immune suppressants, slowing down its natural disease-fighting mechanisms. Ever noticed how you're more prone to colds when you feel under pressure? It's not just your imagination. People in one study were most likely to develop a cold if they had experienced a negative life event in the past year. Another study found that the effectiveness of a pneumonia vaccine was reduced if recipients were suffering from stress.

That's where massage comes in. Regular massage reduces stress and anxiety. It can also boost the immune system by increasing levels of infection-fighting cells. If you don't have a partner or friend you can coerce into giving you a weekly massage, simply get a tennis ball, lean against a wall and roll the ball around between your back and shoulders and the wall.

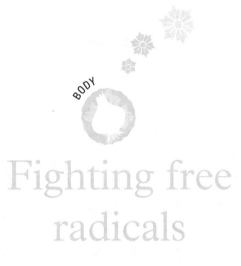

BODY

Fighting free radicals

Free radicals are the body's enemies. Getting rid of them will keep you young and healthy.

If you want a graphic illustration of the power of antioxidants, take an apple, halve it and cover one half of the white flesh with lemon juice. Come back in 30 minutes and the lemon half will be white. That's because it has vitamin C, a prime antioxidant that fights the damage done to the apple by exposure to the air, or oxidation. We need oxygen to enter the bloodstream, combine with carbohydrates and fats to create energy, but the side effect of this is the creation of molecules called oxidants (or free radicals) which roam around the body causing damage. In order to mop them up and 'take them out' we need molecules called antioxidants.

The easiest way to get enough antioxidants is to eat loads of fresh fruit and veg. Choose different colours and eat seasonally to make sure you get a good mixture. The sooner fruits and vegetables are eaten after picking, the more antioxidants they contain. Organic food won't have been left lying around so long, which makes it a good choice. The Okinawans of Japan who have more 105 year olds than anywhere else in earth eat seven to ten servings of fruit and vegetables a day.

Don't add to the free radical load

That means giving up smoking, which loads the body with millions of free radicals every time you inhale. The free radicals in cigarettes cause the fat in your blood to oxidise and form plaques on the artery walls, which is why smokers have a raised risk of heart disease.

Don't sunbathe

Exposure to ultraviolet light floods the skin with free radicals and causes 80–90% of skin ageing.

Exercise regularly

Keep it moderate, though. Great news for anyone who hates painful red-in-the-face exercise sessions, intense exercise uses up large amounts of oxygen and produces similarly large amounts of free radicals as a by-product. The body can't mop up the free radicals quickly enough and damage may occur, which is why athletes can suffer from depressed immune systems. But this isn't carte blanche to become part of the sofa – moderate exercise stimulates the production of the body's antioxidant enzymes and slows the ageing process. Aim for a minimum of around 30 minutes of brisk walking a day.

Boosting your antioxidants

It's easier to do than you might think, thanks to the brilliant scientists at Tufts University in the US, who have very helpfully rated the antioxidant value of every food. It's a system known as ORAC: oxygen radical absorption capacity. The higher the ORAC, the more powerful a food is at mopping up free radicals. In fact, eating plenty of high-ORAC foods could raise the antioxidant power of blood by 10–25%.

One Tufts study of 1300 older people showed that those who had two or more portions a day of dark-pigmented vegetable such as kale and spinach were only half as likely to suffer a heart attack – and had a third of the risk of dying of cancer – compared with people averaging less than one portion a day. Other research has shown that a diet of high-ORAC foods fed to animals prevents long-term memory loss and improves learning capabilities. It may be no coincidence that this high-ORAC diet is very similar to the one eaten by the Hunza people of the Indian Himalayas, who commonly live beyond 100.

The researchers at Tufts think it's the whole foodstuff and the way the hundreds of micronutrients within it (some of which they're yet to identify) react together that provides its powerful antioxidant punch. If you're the cautious type take a belt-and-braces approach, aim for high-ORAC diet and add a good antioxidant supplement just in case.

Top scoring ORAC foods

The following figures are the number of ORACs that 100g
of each food provides. A high-ORAC diet will provide
3000–5000 units a day.

Prunes	5770
Raisins	2830
Blueberries	2400
Blackberries	2036
Garlic	1939
Kale	1770
Cranberries	1750
Strawberries	1540
Spinach	1260
Raspberries	1220
Brussels sprouts	980
Plums	949
Alfalfa sprouts	930
Broccoli	890
Beetroot	840
Avocado	782
Oranges	750
Red grapes	739
Red peppers	710
Cherries	670
Kiwi fruit	602

Baked beans	503
Pink grapefruit	483
Kidney beans	460
Onion	450
White grapes	446

To make the ORAC system work for you, aim to add a handful or two of high ORAC foods to each meal: a handful of prunes or blueberries to your cereal; spinach leaves or avocado into your chicken sandwich; a dish of steamed red cabbage and raisins with your main meal. Carry dried fruit, plums and red grapes as a snack.

You've probably noticed that the ORAC list contains a lot of purple and red foods. Antioxidant compounds are responsible for the bright colour of fruit and vegetables, which is where the 'eat a rainbow' advice comes from. The more deeply coloured the fruit and vegetables the better. We tend to be pretty conservative in our fruit and veg consumption, sticking to just a few. The greatest antioxidant benefit comes from getting the widest variety as possible. Actively look for ways to include as much variety as possible: add carrot and sweet potato to your normal mash; toss a handful of halved baby plum tomatoes when you're frying sausages; grate and add red cabbage to coleslaw.

BODY

Tired or ill?

You're always tired. And now you're beginning to wonder if it could be a sign of something more sinister.

How can you tell the difference between the sort of tiredness that means you've been overdoing it and the sort of tiredness that means you're ill?

Action plan

1. If persistent tiredness is accompanied by pain or unexplained weight loss, you should see your doctor as soon as possible for a check up.
2. Go back to energy basics. The most common causes of exhaustion in young-ish adults is lack of good quality sleep, lack of space in your life, and lack of good food. If you're still tired after two weeks of TLC, see your doctor to explore further possibilities.
3. The two most overlooked causes of unexplained tiredness are reaction to medication (including alternative therapies) – and not realising you're pregnant. Discount both first.

What kind of tired are you?

A gradual onset tiredness that creeps up on you.

Anything else?

Needing to go to the loo more often, excessive thirst, weight loss, genital itching or thrush.

Could be: Diabetes

Diabetes is the disease with a 'silent million' sufferers. A million have it: another million are undiagnosed. It's also a disease on the rise: sedentary lifestyles and an overdependence on processed food are contributing factors and more people than ever in their forties are discovering they've got it. If you are over 40, or you have other risk factors such as a family history or being overweight, your doctor should be happy to test you for diabetes if you suspect if it's at the root of your tiredness.

What kind of tired are you?
   Lethargic and having difficulty concentrating.

Anything else?
   Shortness of breath, dizziness.

Could be: Anaemia

The tissues of your body need oxygen, which is carried to them by the red blood cells. Red blood cells need iron, so a shortage of iron is one cause of anaemia. Menstruating women are most at risk, but anyone can get anaemia, especially if their diet isn't supplying enough iron. Eat more iron-rich foods – red meat, fortified cereals and dried fruit – and take a multivitamin with iron in it. The medical line is that you have to have full-blown anaemia to suffer from chronic tiredness but a study showed that, when iron was given for unexplained tiredness to non-anaemic women, their tiredness diminished. Technically this was the placebo response in action, but the researchers concluded that since many of these non-anaemic women had low blood iron (just enough to be clinical), low-grade iron deficiency could still cause symptoms.

Wash down iron supplying foods with a glass of orange juice: vitamin C helps iron absorption. (Don't take iron supplements without checking with your doctor first.)

What kind of tired are you?
Slow, sluggish, everything in slow motion.

Anything else?
Feeling cold, depression, weight gain, dry thickened skin.

Could be: Hypothyroidism

This is a growing problem and the trouble is not in treatment but in diagnosis. The symptoms start so slowly that often they are misdiagnosed as another disease, for instance, depression or the menopause. If you suspect hypothyroidism, and you're in your 40s or 50s, ask your doctor to test your thyroid hormone levels. Replacement hormones can then be prescribed if a deficiency is found. Younger women may have to exclude other diseases before their doctor is willing to test them.

What kind of tired are you?

Tired all day despite sleeping at night – or perhaps you can't sleep at night. On waking, the thought of the day ahead is exhausting.

Anything else?

Lack of joy and motivation, anxiety, sleep problems, loss of libido, lack of interest in your life, eating too much or too little.

Could be: Depression

Exhaustion is one of the prime symptoms of depression. However, depressed people can help themselves by taking gentle exercise every day. Exercise has been proven to improve mood and it will help you sleep at night – good because insomnia makes you even more isolated. Your GP can help with antidepressants and perhaps by offering counselling and other alternatives to drugs. Phone lines such as the Samaritans can listen for free. There is a wealth of advice available now that the stigma associated with depression is disappearing.

Halle Berry's
health plan

Halle Berry has diabetes, which remained undiagnosed until she collapsed on set in a coma that lasted for seven days. 'I could have gone blind, or lost a limb,' she has said. 'I was terrified.'

She heeded the warning

Halle immediately stopped self-medicating her low blood sugar by eating chocolate bars as she had done before. She started on a diet to balance her blood sugar comprising loads of fresh vegetables, fish, pasta but less fruit because of its high sugar content. She also gave up red meat to help her cholesterol levels.

She took up yoga

Yoga has been shown to help with stress and also helps with diabetes by reducing waist circumference, decreasing blood pressure and blood glucose. Halle practises daily.

She remains positive

'Diabetes turned out to be a gift,' she says. 'It gave me strength and toughness because I had to face reality, no matter how painful or uncomfortable.'

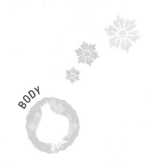

BODY

Just a minute to more energy

One-minute bursts of energy slipped into your usual routine will revolutionise your energy levels.

Just about the fastest way of feeling instantly more energetic is to get the blood pounding in your ears and the breath whizzing in and out of your lungs. A quick burst of activity is also great for dissipating stress hormones. Learning how to navigate through your day, building in little pockets of activity, is a sure way of becoming more stress-resilient and better prepared to meet the demands of your life.

One-minute bursts of activity and slightly longer sessions throughout the day will see your energy levels soar and you can also feel good that you are doing enough to look after your body, too. Research carried out in the US shows that those who are active for 30 minutes three times a week are as healthy as those who exercise at a gym. This idea has been accepted by our own authorities and they recommend being active for 20–30 minutes a day, most days. Being active means gardening, walking briskly to work, climbing stairs rather than using lifts, playing football with the kids and vigorous housework.

If you want more energy

Cast your eye over the following programme and search out the one-minute boosters that appeal to you. Try these or something similar and feel the difference in your energy levels.

If you want to get fit

You need a plan to be sure that you are doing your 30 minutes a day. Here is a sample timetable of how you could build in enough activity.

7 a.m. One-minute booster. Place your alarm clock at the bottom of the bed. Stretch to reach it. Now you've started, don't stop. Spend a minute stretching bed. Movement stimulates the waking part of the brain and makes getting up easier.

7.15 a.m. Ten minutes 'being active'. Do some yoga stretches such as the sun salutation, or some resistance training with some light weights. Increasing blood flow and raising your body temperature will help wake you up.

8 a.m. One-minute booster. While you're waiting for the kettle to boil do star jumps for one minute.

9 a.m. Ten minutes 'being active'. Walk to a newsagent five minutes from your home or desk for your morning paper. There and back equals ten minutes' activity.

11.30 a.m. One-minute booster. While sitting at your desk do some abdominal 'pull-ins'. Sit straight in your chair. Breathe in and bring your navel in and up, hold and let out.

Each one should take a second. Aim for 60 in the morning (and fit in another 60 in the afternoon).

One-minute bursts of activity will see your energy levels soar

1 p.m. Lunch. If you were going to be really good, you could fit in a quick walk, gym visit or run up and down the stairs a few times.

3 p.m. One-minute booster. Stretch out the tension in your shoulders by standing straight and clasping your hands behind your back.

5 p.m. One-minute booster. Get a refreshing drink, say, a green tea. While you're waiting for the kettle to boil, run up and down stairs for one minute.

6 p.m. Ten minutes 'being active'. If you're going to exercise properly this is a good time to do it. If not, do some activity when you get home – gardening or running up and down stairs.

Time for an oil change?

In the last 10 years, there's been an explosion in the research into fats and oils and how much they can benefit our health. It can get confusing – with new advice coming out daily. Here are three basic rules: follow these and you will be maximising your health.

Use more olive oil

Olive oil lowers bad cholesterol and raises good, and it improves digestion. It's also packed with antioxidant vitamins A and E as well as vitamins D and K, vital for strong bones. Those Mediterranean populations where people live the longest use it with abandon – olive oil is poured neat over salads, used on bread rather than butter and drizzled over cooked vegetables.

When shopping stick to extra virgin olive oil. It has the highest concentration of cancer-fighting antioxidants. The other stuff may have had additional treatment or been blended with lesser quality refined oils with some virgin oil added. It won't be as good for you.

Stick to nature's polyunsaturated oils

Polyunsaturated vegetable oils come from natural sources such as nuts and fish, and are essential for a healthy heart and brain. Once they are processed to become oils, their natural antioxidants are removed, and they may even contain side products of the manufacturing process (liquid oxidation products – LOPs) which can attack the arteries. Keep soy, peanut and corn oils to a minimum (often these are just labelled 'vegetable oils'). Sunflower oil is a better choice as it contains higher levels of the antioxidant vitamin E, but the best choice of all, for cooking and dressings, is olive oil.

Avoid trans fats

These are a form of polyunsaturates that are made when oils are processed by hydrogenation. This is used by the food industry to provide moistness in foods such as cakes, biscuits, pastries, pies and sausages. It's also used to stop margarines melting at room temperature and found in many polyunsaturated margarines marketed as 'healthy'.

But they can raise levels of the bad cholesterol in the body to a greater extent than even saturated fats (the kind from animals we're always being told to cut down on). They have been linked to cancer and heart disease. Avoid anything that contains 'hydrogenated vegetable oil', 'trans fats' or 'partially hydrogenated' in the label.

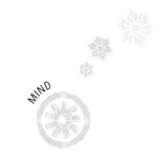

MIND

Avoid the brain drain

Are you feeling mentally sluggish? Having difficulty concentrating? You can revitalise your thinking power in just two weeks.

Brain ageing starts far younger than most of us imagine. How young? Your 20s. No sooner has your brain stopped growing than it starts deteriorating. Ironic? No kidding. But given there's not much mileage in railing against evolution, what can we do about it? Genetics is only about one-third of what determines brain ageing, say the boffins at UCLA's Anti-ageing Institute. The other two-thirds have to do with our environment and lifestyle choices.

Retrain your brain

If you're mentally sluggish and have trouble remembering not just where you left the car keys, but where you left the car, try this programme based on the latest research into brain drain. You can hope to see more mental sharpness within a few weeks.

Every morning

Chuck a handful of blueberries, prunes or raisins onto your cereal or porridge. These and other fruits and vegetables which have a deep-blue colour are particularly high in the 'ORAC' scale and that means they are rich in the brain-boosting anti-ageing antioxidants.

Every day

Eat three meals and two snacks. Your brain needs a steady flow of fuel. Aim for at least one food supplying omega-3 oils – that's avocados, walnuts and, of course, fish. Or pop a supplement – either fish oil, or flaxseed oil, or evening primrose oil if you're a vegetarian. Limit saturated fatty foods: red meat and dairy.

Every couple of hours

De-stress. Cortisol is released when we're stressed and, according to Dr Small from UCLA, who has written several books on keeping your brain active, 'constant stress shrinks a key memory centre [in the brain]. Every hour or so, stand up, take a deep breath and raise your arms above your head. Exhale and drop your arms. Repeat three times. This de-stresses your brain and your body as well as sending oxygen to your brain. Better still, when you are suddenly stressed and flooded with adrenaline, get into the habit of going for a brisk walk as soon as you can. As you know, sitting stewing in a foul mood makes it impossible to think straight – that's because cortisol actually inhibits your brain from working. Moving briskly 'burns off' the cortisol, allowing you to think straight again.

Every two or three days

Go for a walk. Walking every two or three days for 10 minutes, building up to 45 minutes, was found to result in an improvement in mental agility. Stretching and toning exercises did not have this effect.

Are crossword puzzles the answer?

Research shows that the brain can be retrained right into your 80s to learn new languages and skills – or, indeed, how to do crosswords – but University of Virginia research shows that while mental challenges will keep you competent at doing those selfsame mental challenges, they will not necessarily stop Alzheimer's.

But don't throw out your crosswords and computer games yet. You can become sharper at mental challenges by practising. You can make yourself better at thinking quickly or laterally and that is a skill worth having at any age.

You can practise these sort of games at any time. Set yourself a goal such as recalling what your partner was wearing at breakfast; or what the first three people you met this morning said to you. Try to make connections around the numbers in a mobile phone number with the aim of recalling it from memory.

SPIRIT

Try a little tenderness

We're much better at taking care of others than we are of ourselves. But the most important person to start taking care of is you.

Self-care demands much more than the occasional beauty treatment or bout of physical exercise. Self-care is about eating nourishing foods, taking care of your spiritual and emotional well-being, spending quality time with friends and family, or taking yourself away on retreat. No waiting until you've run yourself into the ground or you're running on empty. Your self-care needs to be ongoing and topped up on a regular basis with self-care treats.

It's so easy when you're busy to forget about your self-care rituals. So why not treat yourself as a project? Create a self-care list of ten things that nourish you. Consciously refer to the list when you feel depleted or drained. You're more likely to make better choices about your self-care at that moment than reaching for a handful of crisps or a glass of wine.

If you're struggling to come up with nourishing activities, examining your guilty pleasures may give you some valuable clues. Guilty pleasures are the things you know that if you did more often would make you feel better, but you don't. 'I really could do with a break from the kids but would that make me look bad as a parent?' 'I wish I could have an evening off from the family but I only feel justified to do that if I'm working.' Most of the time you know exactly what you wish you could do to give yourself some *me* time – you just feel guilty about doing it. And herein lies the challenge.

Make a list of all the things you feel bad about wanting to do. Go on. No one has to see your list except you.

A straightforward way of doing this is to turn an everyday routine into a luxury indulgence. There may not be time for a visit to the spa or the funds to book yourself in for a full beauty treatment but that's no reason to put your self-care on hold. A normal bath can be upgraded to a four-star treatment by paying that little bit more for good-quality bath products; adding a few fresh flowers and a tray of candles to give the room that extra special feeling; as you step out of the bath pat yourself dry with an extra large and fluffy bath sheet that has been warmed on a radiator.

Customise your bath

For more bath-time bliss go green in the bathroom by recycling everyday ingredients raided from your kitchen cupboards and fridge that won't cost the earth. One or two tablespoons of ground ginger added to your bath stimulates circulation. Add seven drops of your favourite essential oil and two tablespoons of organic honey into a jug or large bowl of semi-skimmed or organic milk. Warm up in the microwave for three minutes and add it to the bath.

Give yourself the spa treatment before you step into the shower. Polish up dull looking skin by rubbing on a body scrub, starting with the soles of your feet and working your way upwards using circular movements.

For a do-it-at-home facial fill the bathroom sink with warm water and add three drops of lavender essential oil. Soak a warm flannel in the fragrant water then head for the bedroom, lie down, cover your face with the cloth for ten minutes and inhale the aroma.

Putting yourself first is central to living a healthy life. It is counter-intuitive to most women who instinctively care for family first. But remember the metaphor of flying with young children: if there is an emergency, you put on your oxygen mask first so that you can better take care of them. By putting some time aside each week for self-nurturing, you ensure that you have the energy and enthusiasm for others, whilst replenishing your batteries so that you have the focus to get on with your goals and do the things that will help you achieve your success. Taking time to look after yourself as you would anyone else you love will nourish your creativity and help you up your game. Not only that but your self-care will also ensure that you will feel good about you, which gives you energy that can be channelled into your relationships and connections with others. Think of it as being self-full not selfish. It's selfish to deprive ourselves and others of the very best we can be.

Feel good now: *Have an Epsom salts bath. Dissolve 500g or so of Epsom salts (from any chemist) in warm water and relax for 30 minutes. Sip water throughout. Avoid if you have high blood pressure, heart trouble or diabetes. Go straight to bed afterwards. You should sleep like a baby and wake refreshed.*

Two

Making changes

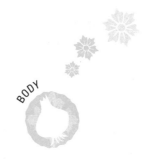

BODY

The real reason you're so tired

The questions below may seem deceptively simple, not to say insulting. But you might find that answering them very quickly pinpoints energy drains that you haven't recognised.

Be honest. Don't check what you know to be the right answers but what you actually do.

1 Do you usually sleep for at least seven and a half to eight hours each night?

2 Do you rarely wake during the night?

3 Do you eat three well-balanced meals a day at regular intervals?

4 Do you always eat breakfast?

5 Do you eat at least two portions of protein foods every day (meat, fish, eggs, dairy, pulses) as well as two portions of wholegrain carbohydrates (bread, pasta or porridge)?

6 Do you eat at least five portions of fruit and vegetables a day?

7 Are you active, on the go for at least an hour a day or more?

8 Do you drink at least one and half litres of fluid a day, not counting very strong coffee, alcohol or energy drinks, and keep you alcohol levels within recommended limits?

9 Do you feel content and happy with your lot?

10 Do you feel that you have a good work–life balance?

Score 2 points for each yes, 0 for each no.

If you scored 16 or over but you feel really lethargic, it might be worth having a chat with your doctor in case there's any underlying medical condition affecting your energy levels, especially if you answered 'no' to question 9. You may have some level of depression. Or you may smoke. (Any and all changes you make to give yourself more energy will be totally undermined by smoking because it adversely affects every single element you need to address in order to be energetic.)

If you scored 10–14. Any single one of these habits can wreak havoc with your energy levels. If you answered 'yes' to questions 1 or 2, your sleep patterns need work; 'yes' to 3–6, your diet doesn't sound as if it's including the basis for providing energy; 'yes' to 7 and you need to think about moving your body more; 'yes' to 9 and 10 and the way you live your life may need an overhaul, or you may be depressed.

If you scored 8 or less. You may be sabotaging yourself on several fronts. Every 'no' is an area you can work at.

Most of us know the basics of what we should do to be healthy, and brimming with energy. These basics are:

- Eating enough good-quality food to provide your cells with energy and keep energy production strong and constant;

- Sleeping enough to restore your body;
- Drinking enough fluids to remain hydrated;
- Exercising enough to keep your lungs and heart functioning healthily and pumping blood to your cells where it supplies the nutrients you need; and
- Stop smoking.

Perhaps you used to do all this. Perhaps you're a mother who just hasn't time to eat properly or exercise, and suffering from sleep disruption; perhaps work has got frantic over the last 6 months and you're so stressed you can't be bothered to look after yourself; perhaps your job demands a lot of travel – if you travel a lot, it's well nigh impossible to take care of the basics unless you put some good systems in place and stick to them until they become habits.

Feel good now: *Don't exercise in the three hours before you go to bed as it can keep you awake. But one study showed that people who do exercise for at least half an hour, four times a week, fall asleep 12 minutes earlier and sleep for 42 minutes longer than people who do no exercise.*

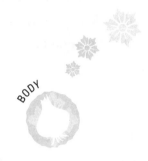

Sleep smarter

If sleep is a problem, remember: it's not just quantity that counts, it's quality. Short sleep breaks can have big calming benefits.

Forget the key to the executive washroom. The latest
perk in the corporate world is the key to the executive
'snoozepod'. Top businesses and even governments
(including the French) are recognising the positive effects
on productivity of having a little nap in the afternoon.

The siesta originated because we all have a natural dip in
alertness in the early afternoon, even if we don't overdo
lunch, and it's especially marked if you've had less sleep the
night before. Most of us reach for a coffee to counteract the
dip but that isn't always the most relaxing solution. Experts
now think we should be reaching for an eye mask and
grabbing forty winks. A 'power nap' revs up your energy
levels for the rest of the day and is worth at least an hour or
so of night-time sleep.

The effects could have to do with the very real power
of a nap to reduce stress levels. Researchers at Harvard
University found a thirty-minute nap could reduce the risk
of burnout, and now we know a nap could save your life –
literally. In a study of thousands of men, it was found that
those who napped in the afternoon were 34% less likely to
get heart disease. The effects were more pronounced in the
men who worked (and had the most stress), so researchers
think that the beneficial effects of a nap are about stress
reduction. Certainly a nap of 15–20 minutes allows the

body to 'cut off' and cell repair to begin. Your brain has time to disconnect and this allows restorative action to take place. When you wake, you feel more alert, have better concentration, and your reactions are quicker.

Winston Churchill, a world-class napper, believed a nap wasn't beneficial unless you got undressed and into bed. Not all of us have that luxury. But you can probably find somewhere comfy to put your head down for a short while. Set a timer to go off in 20 minutes' time, close your eyes, and relax. If you can't sleep, just resting with your eyes closed is enough to give some benefits.

Remember:

• Nap between 2 p.m. and 4 p.m., the natural energy dip.
• Don't nap after 6 p.m. or it could affect your sleep later that night.
• A few minutes daily is better than a longer nap once a week. Little and often is what works the magic. Research in Australia discovered that 10-minute mini-naps increased alertness and productivity, but longer than 20 minutes left participants groggy due to 'sleep inertia' – the sluggishness that occurs when a deep sleep is interrupted.

- At night, if you have trouble drifting off to sleep, the prime reason is probably anxiety. Read a boring book, eat lettuce sandwiches (lettuce and white bread are sleep-inducing) or keep a pad by your bed to write all your random thoughts down so they're out of your head and on the pad. As a last resort, get up and don't go back to bed until you're already half asleep and absolutely sure that you will drop off. Sometimes lying on the floor or the couch will be enough to allow you to drift off. You may be a sufferer of 'psychophysiological insomnia' which means you can fall asleep but just not in bed. The main thing is to ensure that you don't begin to associate your bed with feelings of frustration. Aim to fall asleep fairly easily anywhere – a couch, the floor – and when you get back into a rhythm of dropping off again, start gradually moving back into your bed.

Feel good now: *Get to bed by 9.30 every night for a week. Even if you can't sleep, listen to the radio, soothing music, audiobooks or read. Resting your body helps restore energy.*

Step-by-step napping

- If you're working in an office, switch your phone to voicemail and either sit at your desk or find an empty room. Explain to any line managers what you're up to, that it will increase your productivity and that it will be 20 minutes maximum. Offer to take it off your lunch hour if necessary.
- Find somewhere quiet.
- Loosen your clothing and take off your shoes. Lie down on a sofa, stretch out on the floor or if that's not possible sit comfortably on a chair, placing your head in your folded arms on your desk.
- Close your eyes – ideally put on an eyemask.
- Try not to think about work or all the things you have to do. Focus on what you love doing in your spare time. If you like golf, you might mentally play a round of gold on your regular course. Maybe drift back to a favourite holiday, or listen to some calming music.

- Just rest at first – if your brain needs a rest as well, you'll soon fall asleep.
- Set the alarm to go off in 20 minutes' time, in case you do fall asleep. Don't sleep for more than 30 minutes, you'll wake up groggier and foggier.
- When you wake up lie still for a minute or two – then stretch and breathe deeply and take a drink of water or a light snack to get your system going again. Then return to work, starting with simple chores such as opening letters or planning. Within just a few minutes you should feel sparky again.

Makeover your metabolism

Want to have more energy and lose weight?
Read on.

Strap a couple of laptops round your middle and you'll soon find just how draining carrying around that extra 10lbs can be. If you're overweight, losing a few pounds will help your energy levels. But how do you do it without feeling more drained? Try this: it's called calorie cycling. Versions of it have been around for years but for some reason it isn't trumpeted by the slimming industry. Maybe because it works, and is probably one of the unconscious strategies that naturally slim people operate without realising it. One day you eat a lot and then you take a couple of days or so to recover, eating only lightly. Then you have another binge. Then you take a few days to recover.

Feel good now: *Dieting makes us depressed. Serotonin – the feel-good hormone – dropped much faster in women than men who dieted for three weeks during a University of Oxford study. Your body can't make serotonin without the amino acid tryptophan, and carbohydrate is needed so that tryptophan can reach the brain from the bloodstream. Avoid very low carbohydrate diets.*

Consciously putting calorie cycling into action has the advantage of being realistic. It takes into account that none of us can stick to a diet all the time. Of course, some people do spend their lives on a diet – stick-thin celebs are the most visible example. But if they ever slip up, they will balloon overnight because constant starvation has lowered their metabolic rate – the rate at which they burn off calories – to that of a hedgehog.

Calorie cycling works on the principle that by mixing up your calorie count, your metabolic rate stays on its toes, so to speak. Your metabolic rate doesn't drop as you lose weight; in fact, it revs up. It's thought that dieting suppresses production of an appetite-regulating hormone, leptin. High leptin production means a high metabolism; reduced leptin means metabolism goes down and your appetite goes up. This mechanism helped our stone age ancestors cope with famine. Now it just makes us fat.

How does calorie cycling work? Simple. You diet for a few days, then for one day you eat pretty much what you like. There is evidence that it works. Research done by the National Institute of Health in the United States discovered that when healthy young men restricted calories and then binged, their metabolism rose by 9% on the morning after their binge day; it's thought binge days reset leptin production.

The hardcore version

This version means you eat lightly during the day (but frequently), and more at night. You further mix things up by dropping most carbs for a couple of days then adding them back in. The advantage is that you are never more than three days away from pudding. Eat unlimited amounts of fruit and salad during the day with eggs as your only protein. At night, eat unlimited amounts of vegetables with a large-ish piece of protein – beef, chicken, turkey, fish, or tofu. Don't eat any starch or sugars.

If you're overweight, losing a few pounds will help your energy levels

Follow this for two days then switch to one day of eating much the same, but, after you've eaten your evening meal, have some carbohydrates – a roll, a baked potato, some pasta or rice and a dessert, too, if you like. You must eat the protein and vegetables first because the theory goes that you should never eat starchy carbohydrate foods on an empty stomach. The sugars are rapidly absorbed into your bloodstream resulting in a blood-sugar spike and release of insulin, which encourages your body to store excess energy as fat. Eating non-starchy carbs such as vegetables and protein beforehand slows down the absorption of sugars.

The straightforward version

Eat around 1700 calories for four or five days. Eat around 2000 calories for one day. Eat 1700 calories for four or five days. Eat around 2000 calories for one day. You get the picture. Don't do this for more than a month because it is low in calories.

The simplest version

Stick to a low-calorie, low-carb or low-fat diet of your choice for six days and eat what you like on the seventh. You will probably go mad for the first few weeks on your free day, and then you will relax into it. Eat a bit more, enough for calorie cycling to work, but on the whole eat healthily.

The danger

The big problem with calorie cycling is if you slip up and have more days 'off' than 'on'. This means you may put weight on. As a rule of thumb, never have more than two days 'off' in a row. If you can't trust yourself to break a diet and then go back on it again, this isn't the scheme for you.

What 1700 calories looks like

- Breakfast – bowl of cereal with semi-skimmed milk and a small glass of orange juice
- Mid-morning – half a dozen almonds
- Lunch – sandwich, apple
- Mid-afternoon – orange
- Dinner – chicken and vegetable stir-fry followed by a peach and a small glass of wine.

Quiz:
Is your problem too much adrenaline?

You're firing on all cylinders, dealing with crisis after crisis. You feel that you're in fifth gear while everyone else is pootling along in third.

You are coping brilliantly, the trouble is no one else is. Everyone else is driving you mad and you're constantly irritable. That's because although it feels as if you are making decisions at lightning speed, multitasking brilliantly, you're running on adrenaline and you're stressed out almost permanently.

1 **While you were eating breakfast this morning you were:**
   a) Sitting at the table, or in bed, listening to the radio.
   b) Running around blowdrying your hair or on the way to work.
   c) Breakfast is for wimps.

2 **When you are deciding where to eat a lunch, you choose:**

a) The nicest place you can afford.

b) The nearest place to your desk, indeed, most often at your desk.

c) Lunch is for wimps.

3 **What were you doing this time last week?**

a) Give me a second and I can tell you.

b) It's a bit of a blur.

c) Why would I waste my time even thinking about it?

4 **When you're forced to wait for a red light, a train or in a queue at the bank, you:**

a) Daydream happily.

b) Get fidgety.

c) Start hyperventilating.

5 **When you're watching a DVD, you're feeling:**

a) Absorbed in the drama – you use it to relax.

b) Guilty – you should be doing something more productive.

c) Driven to tears. Why do the characters talk so slowly? Couldn't the director get them to pick up the pace?

6 Do you find yourself finishing people's sentences?

a) Never, awfully rude.

b) Yes, when you know the people well.

c) All the time. You've worked out what you're going to say before they have.

If you scored mostly as – you're calm and safe from overdrive.

If you scored mostly bs – watch out for stress levels, they're on the rise.

If you scored a mixture of bs and cs – you're running your life almost entirely on adrenaline. You need to slow down fast.

BODY

Improving your digestion

Good health starts with good digestion. An inefficient bowel leads to disease. Understanding how it works is the first step.

An important measure of bowel performance is transit time – how long it takes from the time you eat a food until it comes out the other end. The most effective way to measure this is to eat three or four whole beetroots. Beetroot turns the stools red: if you take note of when you eat the beets you can calculate how long your own personal transit time is. (Sweetcorn works well, too.) Twelve to twenty-four hours is the optimal transit time. If it's less than 12 hours, it's possible you're not absorbing all the nutrients you should be from your food. More than 24 hours indicates that the waste is sitting in your insides for too long and this can greatly increase the risk of colon disease.

How do you increase your transit time?

* Increase fibre. Up the amount of fruit, vegetables and pulses. Whole grains are also full of fibre. Whole grains are unprocessed grains where the husk and fibre hasn't been removed. That's why brown rice is much better for you than white. Not all brown bread is wholegrain. Some is merely dyed so that it looks healthier. If it's light and airy, it's unlikely to be that healthy. Look for the word 'wholemeal' on the label.
* Increase water intake.

- Watch for foods that react negatively in the gut. These include sugar, alcohol, high-fat foods and processed foods like chips, pastries and ready-made meals.
Foods which contain flour are particularly able to slow everything down. Remember making glue from flour and water at primary school? The same thing goes on in your gut.

You have around 4lbs of bacteria in your digestive system. Among these trillions of bacteria are the goodies that help you resist food poisoning, protect you against disease and make minerals and vitamins available to the body. To increase their number, eat cultured foods such as yoghurt, sauerkraut and cottage cheese. Or you could take a daily supplement with live bacteria in it (just one tablet can be the equivalent of 15 small tubs of yoghurt).

Watch out for stress

Part of the 'fight or flight' syndrome involves the digestive system shutting down. So if you are frequently stressed, your bowel function could well be erratic. Digestive enzymes can help (consult a nutritionist). Or reduce stress, of course!

A six-week plan to transform your energy levels

Each week, concentrate on adding in one habit. You can do them all at once but, if you find eating regularly and well a challenge, take it one week at a time.

1 Eat breakfast. Every day.
2 Eat lunch. Every day.
3 Start snacking. Never go longer than three hours without eating. Regular healthy snacks mean you don't overeat at meal times. Since eating huge amounts at mealtimes can deplete your energy – about 10% of your daily energy intake goes on digesting what you eat, and a big meal means you're doing it all at once. Snacking is less stressful for your body. It also keeps your blood-sugar levels stable so you have a constant flow of energy throughout the day.

4 Add in energy-giving carbs. Eat a fist-sized portion of wholegrain carbohydrates at every meal because it supplies B vitamins and doesn't get broken down too fast: for instance, wholegrain pasta, brown rice, oats or wholemeal bread (around two slices). Wholegrain contains fibre and fibre slows down release of the sugars in carbohydrates into the bloodstream. This means a slow release of energy throughout the day.

5 Add in energy-giving protein. Eat a deck of cards-sized portion of protein at lunch – and if you really want to see a difference in your energy levels, have some at breakfast too. That means meat, fish, eggs (× 2), cottage cheese, cheese, tofu.

6 Drink enough fluid – about one to two litres a day – not including alcohol or strongly caffeinated drink.

Michelle Pfeiffer's
health plan

She believes she's in charge of her destiny

A fat child, who was bullied and teased, Michelle showed great determination and focus in turning around her eating and exercising habits and losing a lot of weight while still very young.

She believes in moderation

'I eat well but at my age I'll say "what the hell" and have a Krispy Kreme. To make up for it, I sprint, go hiking and do daily Pilates. You have to work out if you want to eat.'

She loves organic

She only uses organic skin care products and her own chef travels with her when she's abroad to ensure her diet is wholesome and healthy. Every morning she has a smoothie for breakfast made from white peaches and red berries for their antioxidant value.

She doesn't fret about what she can't change

'I don't think about ageing,' she says. 'There's no way you can stop it. You can all have the surgeries you want, but you're still getting older.'

Shopping for energy

Turn your supermarket shop into an energy-boosting adventure.

Live a little – eat more! Choosing from a wide variety of foods will boost your energy.

The average woman eats only around 20 different foods. Nutritionists say that we should eat from the widest variety of foods possible because unsurprisingly, that will result in getting the optimal number of nutrients. You should be looking to make your choice from between 60 to 70 different foods on a regular basis.

There are two advantages when it comes to your energy levels in mixing it up.

• You will be eating a cornucopia of energy-boosting nutrients.
• You will render your shopping trips a lot more interesting.

The nutrients that are vital for energy release are the B vitamins, vitamin C, magnesium, iron and chromium. Shopping with the following lists in mind will ensure you're getting enough of them.

The top ten multi-taskers

To make it really easy when you're shopping *add three of these a week* to your shopping trolley and mix it up: select another three next week. They have been chosen to supply a good mix of B vitamins, magnesium, iron and chromium.

1 Bran Flakes or All-Bran – packed with iron, B vitamins and vitamin C.
2 Beef – iron, chromium (liver is good, too).
3 Wholegrain rice and bread – B vitamins and magnesium.
4 Chick peas – magnesium and iron.
5 Oats – B vitamins and magnesium.
6 Sardines – magnesium and iron.
7 Quorn – loaded with key B vitamins.
8 Turkey – vitamin B12 and iron.
9 Nuts and seeds – mix and match different types for 'broad spectrum' cover. Pumpkin seeds are a particularly good source of iron.
10 Rye bread – good for iron and B vitamins.

Twelve brilliant sources of vitamin C

Choose three a week on top of your normal foodstuffs and mix them up every week.

These all supply more than 20mg per 100 g of Vitamin C.

1 Blackcurrants.

2 Bran Flakes.

3 Brussels sprouts.

4 Cabbage (raw has double).

5 Cauliflower.

6 Citrus fruits.

7 Kiwi fruit.

8 Mango.

9 Red and orange peppers (raw).

10 Raspberries.

11 Strawberries.

12 Watercress.

Six top snacks

These combine the all-important energy combo: protein with carbohydrate. Stock up with enough of these so that when you need a between-meal-pick-me-up, you can reach for a snack that will fill you up without sending your blood sugar soaring (which leads to a slump in energy later). Some of these may seem a bit odd at first, but just try them mid-morning and mid-afternoon and you'll be amazed at how satisfied you'll feel.

1 Two oatcakes with peanut butter.

2 Nuts – a good handful with a few sultanas or cranberries if you like.

3   A stick of celery spread with cream or cottage cheese.
4   Slices of apple spread thinly with peanut or other nut butter.
5   A vegetable juice with a few nuts on the side.
6   A boiled egg and couple of rye crispbreads or a slice of rye bread.

Other great foods to add to your shopping list on a regular basis

Eggs (protein/vitamin B); mackerel (best source of omega-3); bulgur (good source of slow-releasing carb for long-lasting energy); Marmite (B vitamins); basil (beloved by herbalists for its uplifting qualities); artichoke (vitamin C and magnesium); beetroot (high in vitamin C, magnesium, iron and B vitamins); kale (packed with iron and B vitamins); lentils (loaded with magnesium); celery (has special phytochemicals that are good for energy and improving mood).

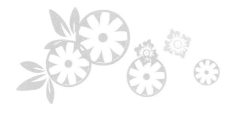

Eat with the calendar

Another good way to ensure you get a good mix of phytochemicals nutrients and also to liven up your shopping is to eat foods in season. Try a new recipe at least once every month that uses seasonal foods.

January: turnips, scallops, parsnips
February: chicory, celeriac, cabbage
March: rhubarb, radishes, purple sprouting broccoli
April: lamb, rosemary, spinach
May: asparagus, broad beans, cherries
June: strawberries, gooseberries, courgettes
July: blueberries, fennel, aubergines
August: greengages, basil, peppers
September: damsons, plums, autumn lamb
October: figs, elderberries, watercress
November: chestnuts, beetroot, cranberries
December: pomegranates, red cabbage, celery

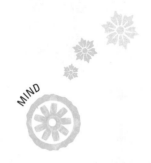

MIND

Getting over being overwhelmed

Got too much to handle? Having problems keeping on top of your work? Here's how to prioritise so you can spend more time on the things you really want to do.

In an ideal world most people would love to prioritise tasks and projects based on what they deem as important. But in real life most of us operate in the opposite way.

We prioritise based on urgency, which falls down to the fact that by the time a task is urgent, it's often too late to do a good job on it: we don't give ourselves enough time to get tasks completed on time without half killing ourselves.

Bitten off more than you can chew?

One way to avoid the stress of having to prioritise in the first place is to get on top of handling a task or project as soon as you receive it. So let's say you have a report to produce in one month's time and you want to avoid getting to a place where writing the report is deemed as urgent. Take the approach of getting started on the report almost right away. This is not something to think on but rather to do. So the request for the report comes in via an email. Decide you'll devote 15 minutes to it every day for the next week, and after a week decide whether you need to up the amount of time each day you are spending on it. Within the next 24 hours schedule a space in your day where you can grab 15 minutes and brainstorm a list of the contents of the report. The next day you might write a rough draft of the introduction. On day three you might spend your 15 minutes beginning research. Keep this approach going over the next three weeks, increasing the amount of time you spend on it as the deadline grows closer.

In real life most of us prioritise based on urgency

If you are bamboozled by the sheer volume that you have to do on a task, write a list of five things that you absolutely have to do, and start on one of them.

You'll notice that you'll feel more in control and far less stressed. Producing work driven by a sense of urgency on a regular basis puts you in danger of producing work that's average and poor quality.

The other side of this is to be careful of falling prey to allowing yourself to be dumped on by other people's urgent tasks: tasks that have become urgent because they didn't act sooner. Get into a habit of saying no and giving the responsibility back to the other person. You could say something like, 'I appreciate that this is urgent but if I had received this two weeks ago I would have been able to take action on it sooner.'

Feel good now: *Research shows that popping bills in your bag to pay later subtly stresses you out all day and drains energy. File them or deal with them immediately.*

Inside the box

Get creative and take inspiration from the choreographer and dancer Twyla Tharp, who starts every dance piece with a box. On the box she writes the project name and fills it up with each item that goes into the making of that dance. This includes notebooks, clippings, CDs, videos, books and photos. Over a period of time she places in that box anything that inspires her around the project. She builds in time for research, for reflection and allows herself time and space to experiment.

Your box might be your notebook or a file on your computer. Or notes in a file. It really doesn't matter; what does matter is that you engage with it by beginning the process by creating space.

SPIRIT

Getting to know your shadow

Everyone has a shadow side, parts of our personalities and our character that we've judged as bad or not good. Normal instinct is to hide this part of our personality away from others and ourselves.

But doing the opposite and embracing the shadow may be the ticket to your emotional freedom.

No one's perfect. We all have parts of our personality that we tend to keep hidden. The challenge begins when we've attached certain feelings like shame and humiliation to certain parts of our personality and make-up. The trick is not to do what you've always done, which is to push the shadow self away. Instead practise facing your shadow, embracing it and then finding a way to integrate the shadow with the intention of reducing its overall charge.

Individuals who are comfortable within their own skins are comfortable with all aspects of who they are. The challenge is to keep finding ways of bridging the gap between who you are in your private, secret self and the reputation of your public, open self. It may not be possible to ever fully get rid of the shadow but by recognising it you can certainly change the way the shadow shows up and operates in your life.

These exercises will help you identify aspects of your own shadow and will help you to shift the focus and nature of your shadow self. It's a good idea to capture your responses in your journal as you will need to reflect on these exercises over time.

The Johari window

The Johari window, a self-awareness model, was devised by two psychologists, Joseph Luft and Harry Ingram, back in the 1950s. Draw a large square and divide it into four equal-sized squares. Label the top left-hand box the public self; the bottom left-hand box is the secret self; the top right-hand box the open self; and the box below is the unknown self. The public self comprises the parts others know about us but we're not aware of. The secret self is what we know about ourselves that others don't. The open self consists of the parts others know and we know about in equal proportion, and the unknown self represents the parts of ourselves we are still yet to know.

We all have parts of our personality that we tend to keep hidden

The idea of the Johari window is to decrease the size of the public and secret self through self-disclosure and communication with others that will extend the areas of the open self and ultimately make us more aware of what's in the unknown self. Think about parts of the secret self that you could reveal to those close to you; this would increase intimacy in your relationships. Do you know someone whose opinion you trust whom you could ask to reveal parts of your public self, how you are perceived by others that you might not be aware of? This can help you gain valuable insight and increase the information in the open self.

There really is something wrong with you

What about valuing and accepting your imperfect self, flaws and all? Everyone has flaws, from your doting parents, who in your eyes never put a foot wrong, to the mentor you credit for turning your career around. The problem starts when we judge these aspects of our personality as bad or wrong. Make a list of all your supposed faults. Now remember times when those very traits were useful to you. Bad-tempered? But sometimes that's served you by meaning you don't waste time doing what you don't like. Timid? But that has kept you safe on numerous occasions. You stick your head in the sand? Yes, but often problems simply disappear and you haven't wasted time worrying for no reason.

Mirror, mirror on the wall

By not embracing the imperfect self you run the risk of turning the tables round and homing in on those very same traits in others. What we deny in ourselves we often very quickly notice and dislike in others. And the more cross we are with another, the greater the chance that we are ignoring something within. The old saying 'when we're pointing the finger at another, our thumb is pointing back at us' really is true.

> *When we're pointing the finger at another, our thumb is pointing back at us*

Make a list of all the things – no matter how small – that annoy or irritate you about other people. Now be honest. Can you think of even one time when you could have been

accused of that fault yourself, but perhaps manifesting in a different way? Perhaps you are furious because your partner does what he wants without referring to you, but are you guilty of not listening to him properly? Hint: the behaviour in others which has the most emotional charge for us is usually a sign that we are recognising something in ourselves that we really don't like and would prefer to keep hidden.

Three

Healthy and energised

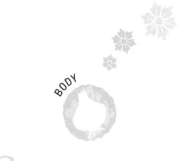

BODY

Stress-proof your health

The good news is that women have hormonal help in coping with stress. The bad news is that this may not be enough to counteract our increasingly stressful lives. So what can you do about it?

Women's brains respond differently to psychological stress and it could be a factor in protecting us from health problems. When we feel stressed, we experience the 'fight or flight' response – we get aggressive or get out of the situation. But following the rush of stress hormones, the posterior pituitary gland releases oxytocin. This counteracts the stress hormones and promotes nurturing feelings, and it would appear to be the reason for the 'tend and befriend' response which predominates in women: when we get stressed we look for support and offer support in return (which is why your phone bill soars when you or your friend is having a bad time). Men get some oxytocin, too, but nothing like as much as women and this means that the stress hormones are relatively unimpeded and eventually leads to hardening of their arteries and heart disease. Scientists now believe that our healthier oxytocin response could be the reason women live on average seven years longer than men.

But we can't afford to be complacent. Stress effects are cumulative, and the evidence is that for many women being stressed practically 24/7 is a way of life. That has big effects on our health. Here is how to stress-proof your body against the effects of twenty-first century life.

Stress-proof your fertility ...

Stress hormones are made in the pituitary, as are the sex hormones, so it's not surprising that they impact one another. Chronic stress increases testosterone production and can eventually affect periods' frequency. It also worsens conditions such as polycystic ovary syndrome which are implicated in infertility but not always picked up until a woman tries to get pregnant.

Common sense response to stress

Start by finding just 20 minutes a day to be still with no noise – a long bath, a break ensconced in a deckchair in the garden, lying in the park during your lunch hour. That's a real challenge for a lot of us these days given that we live by our BlackBerry and iPod, but it really could make a difference to your ability to conceive when you want to.

The other important factor is diet. Start following the dietary recommendations in this book as soon as possible. Cut down on alcohol and, of course, smoking.

Stress-proof your healthy habits

Women who work long hours are more likely than men to eat high-fat and high sugar snacks, exercise less and drink more caffeine, according to a study carried out at the University of Leeds. Men aren't so self-destructive. Why?

It appears women feel that they have less time and also are more home-focused than men. The combination is lethal. A woman worried about getting dinner on the table is likely to forgo a swim at the end of the day and head for home. A study found that women under stress eat less healthily because they don't think they have enough time to eat well.

Common sense response to stress

Be prepared. Don't drift towards the vending machine because you forgot breakfast and need a sugar rush. Make sure you have some healthy nuts and fruit or crudités in your bag. Refuse to forgo your gym session at lunchtime unless it's a genuine emergency. Start making the connection between the role stress plays in making you feel that there's just no time to look after yourself and you'll see ways to guard against your good intentions being sabotaged.

Stress-proof your metabolism

Stress can make you fat. Studies have demonstrated that chronic stress causes our cells to be bathed in cortisol more or less continuously and this changes our ability to produce insulin which leads directly to abdominal obesity. Another way stress makes us fat is that we 'comfort eat': stress makes us desire more high-sugar, high-fat food.

Common sense response to stress

As well as being prepared as outlined above, take breaks throughout your day to sip green tea. It helps your body regulate insulin release. Research is ongoing at the University of Nottingham to discover if green tea's high catechin content helps combat abdominal fat, as has been indicated by previous studies.

Stress-proof your mental health

Women in the UK are twice as likely as men to suffer from depression. We are also more prone to obsessive-compulsive disorder and anxiety conditions.

Research is still preliminary but it appears that the feel-good hormone, serotonin, is affected by oestrogen in a complex interaction in the brain, making us more prone to mood swings, for one thing.

Common sense response to stress

Use your 'tend and befriend' tendencies. Ask friends for feedback? Are you worrying more than usual or giving off a negative 'vibe'? Monitoring your mental outlook – either on your own or via friends – can help us see potential problems coming from a long way away. Looking for help early on can make a big difference to the outcome.

BODY

Safeguard your fertility

How can you maximise your chances of conceiving when you decide you want to start a family?

Do not be terrified by the scare stories. Most women (still) have a baby when they decide they want one, or shortly afterwards. However, there are challenges to our fertility that our mothers didn't face. Young women drink much more and it's thought that they'll find that, for a significant proportion, caning it through their 20s will have an effect on their long-term fertility. But the most obvious challenge is good contraception that means we can start having a family much later. If for you this contraception is a blessing, and you don't want a baby yet but want to ensure that you maximise your chances that you can, what can you do?

The secret is to help your body reproduce cells as efficiently and correctly as possible. This won't just improve your fertility, it will help you stay young, too. Imagine yourself ten years older but looking more or less as you do now (or better). That's what you are aiming for.

Nurture your body so you age slowly

Take folic acid and antioxidant supplements including vitamin E and selenium. Make sure you eat plenty of nuts, seeds, parsley, spinach and asparagus for their high zinc content.

Drink litres of water (at least 2) as apparently water is a crucial element in cell reproduction, whereas caffeine allows mistakes in cell replication to be 'overlooked' by the body.

Consider glyconutrients – these are forms of sugar that are vital in promoting intercellular communication and are thought to help fight off degenerative diseases. Glucose and lactose are pretty ubiquitous but the others are hard for us to come by in our diet. You might want to think of taking supplements (available online) that contain them.

Water is a crucial element in cell reproduction

Limit stress

One large German study found that around 25% of all cases of infertility could be due to stress. In another study of women who were not conceiving, the women were divided into three groups: one group received counselling; one group formed a support group and the third had no intervention. The rates of successful conception in the first two groups was around 55%: in the control group it was around 20%. Start taking steps now to get on top of stress. Having strategies in place now is a lot easier than when you're desperate for a baby and well-meaning friends keep telling you to relax.

Take your sexual health seriously

Arrange to have tests for chlamydia and other sexually transmitted diseases. If you do not use condoms, you should have these tests regularly as many STDs do not have symptoms in many women, so your fertility could be under attack without you ever realising it.

Watch your weight

Weigh yourself and then check your Body Mass Index (BMI) on one of the tools online. If your BMI is less than 20, you might be too thin to conceive. Similarly if it's over 30, you are definitely overweight and should lose some weight; 28–29 and you may well be too heavy. If you are between 25–27, losing a little so that you are somewhere between 20–24, the optimum.

Forget any sort of drug

The less you smoke or take recreational drugs, the more fertile you will be. These certainly affect your ability to conceive if you are still taking them, and it's thought that we will discover that regular use hinders conception even if you give up years before. Alcohol affects DNA, too, although unless you drink unwisely, drying out when you are trying to conceive should mean that you're OK. Keep alcohol consumption at safe levels.

Turning veggie

Studies show that vegetarians live longer and suffer less heart disease and cancer. Is it time to ditch the meat?

If you're a vegetarian, you can afford to feel smug. You're already a winner when it comes to anti-ageing. You can look forward to ten extra years of disease-free living than meat-eaters and you're 39% less likely to die from cancer. You're also 30% less likely to die of heart disease. Studies of the world's longest-lived communities back this up. A study of rural Chinese people who were mainly vegetarian proved that they remained disease-free far longer than their meat-eating urban counterparts who succumb to heart disease, stroke, osteoporosis, diabetes and cancer.

The human race did evolve as omnivores, designed to eat anything. But back all those thousand of years ago, we ate meat rarely: now we eat more meat in a week than our ancestors did in months. There's a theory that humans have a long colon, like a horse or cow, and a relatively slow food transit designed to break down grains and grasses. Too much meat introduced into the system literally rots before it reaches the end, releasing toxins into the bloodstream, and some prominent experts have estimated that around 80–90% of degenerative disease such as cancer and cardiovascular disease could be prevented at least into very old age if we stuck to a plant-based diet.

Meat is, of course, a great source of protein. We need around 35g of protein a day (most meat-eating women are getting around 65g) but we can get it from fish, lentils, beans, grains like rice, quinoa and bulgar wheat, eggs, yoghurt, cheese, nuts, or seeds.

See meat as a treat

If this is all whistling in the wind because you know there's no way you can give up your Sunday roast, then don't despair. Omnivores who eat above average amounts of fruit and vegetables can cut their risk of most cancers by 50–75%. By increasing the amount of plant food you eat, you'll probably find you naturally cut back on meat consumption.

Another way is to see meat as a treat. In Mediterranean countries, red meat is only eaten a couple of times a month on average. Skinless turkey breast is one of the leanest meats available and it's a good source of cancer-fighting selenium and zinc. If you can afford it, opt for organic meat which doesn't contain growth hormones and antibiotics: it is more expensive but if you eat meat just once a week, but go for better quality, it evens out.

The very worst options are processed meats such as hot dogs, burgers and cured meats as they contain high amounts of nitrates which are thought to be carcinogenic. (In one study of 30,000 women, those who ate lot of hamburgers had twice the normal risk of certain kinds of cancer.)

Supplementary benefits

What supplements give you the most bang for your buck in the living younger for longer stakes?

How many times have you read that a healthy, balanced diet should provide all the vitamins and minerals a body needs, and that supplements are a waste of money? In theory, it sounds reasonable. But it doesn't explain why virtually every anti-ageing researcher and scientist takes supplements on a regular basis.

Let's face it, we never quite live up to our healthy intentions. We know we need a minimum of five portions of fruit and veg a day (ten would be better), but average consumption is just about half that. On top of this, certain lifestyle factors such as smoking, drinking, pollution and stress can deplete our body of nutrients. Stress takes its toll on B vitamins, which are required to keep the nervous system healthy. Smoking and drinking leach away vitamin C. Plus, as we age, we require fewer calories on a daily basis, and so our chances of getting the right amount of nutrients from food are reduced. Add to that the fact that modern farming and food processing techniques have reduced the vitamin and mineral content of many foods and you can see the problem.

But what supplements should you take? Here is a simple four-step guide:

1   Start with a daily multivitamin/mineral supplement.
    This will make up for deficiencies caused by trace
    elements missing from your diet. You don't have to
    spend a fortune. Look for a multivitamin that includes
    selenium – a mineral needed in trace amounts that's
    thought to boost the immune system and fight disease.
    One study found that 100 micrograms of selenium
    taken daily reduced the death rate among cancer
    patients. Ideally, your supplement should also include
    around 50mg of magnesium, which helps to lower
    blood pressure.

2   Boost your vitamin C. Vitamin C's main job is to enter
    your cells and lie in wait to eliminate opportunist free
    radicals looking to damage your DNA. It also helps
    heal artery walls that have become damaged, reduce
    cholesterol and lower blood pressure. It's also vital
    for boosting the immune system and plays a big role
    in fighting cancer. Making sure you eat some citrus
    food or berries every day is essential, so add a vitamin
    C supplement of up to 1000mg a day – the current
    recommended safe upper limit. Some anti-ageing
    experts recommend taking up to 3000mg a day,
    although it has been known to cause diarrhoea in high
    doses. Try starting with two daily 500mg doses, six
    hours apart.

3   Boost your vitamin E. Vitamin E can lower the risk of heart attack in women by as much as 40%. If vitamin E is given to people who already show signs of heart disease, it can reduce the risk of heart attack by as much as 75%. In an ideal world, vitamin E likes to work with vitamin C – they complement each other as E is fat-soluble and C is water-soluble, so between them, they've got the body covered. Make sure you're eating wholegrain versions of foods such as cereals, bread, rice or pasta several times a day and green leafy vegetables at least once a day. Then add a supplement of up to 540mg a day.

4   Boost your B_5. Homocysteine is an amino acid which builds up in the blood as you age. Now scientists are linking high homocysteine levels with a higher risk of heart disease. But simply taking a supplement of 400mg of folic acid every day is usually all you need to substantially reduce your homocysteine to safe levels. Folic acid is a B vitamin that likes to work synergistically with the other Bs, so look for a B complex supplement.

Quiz:
Do you take time to recreate?

It's called recreation for a good reason. It's the chance for you to recreate yourself from a stressed out version of you, to the more Zen version that you and everyone else loves. But is there time for that in your schedule?

1 **You're invited to an event that you think will be pretty dire. However, the really good friend inviting you really wants you to go. You:**

   a) Say yes but feel irritated with yourself afterwards for not being able to say no.

   b) Say yes – you can arrive late, you don't have to stay long. There's always time to fit something else in.

   c) Say no – you just don't have time for this sort of thing.

2 **You've had a busy day and a friend phones up for a good moan. You:**
   a) Listen dutifully, you'd feel guilty if you didn't.
   b) Listen for as long as you can but you haven't too long before you have to go out.
   c) Let the answer machine pick it up – you don't have energy for friends in the evening.

3 **You have friends coming for dinner but you've had a hell of a day and don't have time to cook. You:**
   a) Spend a fortune buying food from a deli, and all night apologising for not cooking from scratch.
   b) Send out for a takeaway – your friends know what you're like and half expect it.
   c) Cancel. You just can't face it.

4 **You often feel disappointed:**
   a) In yourself, that you don't get everything done that you'd like to.
   b) That you don't have enough time to see all your friends more regularly or spend enough quality time with family.
   c) That all you seem to do is work.

5 Your friends would say that you:

a) Are often harassed but always there for them.

b) Are often late but do your best to be there for them.

c) Elusive these days – you're always working.

Mostly a) – you are busy because you have free floating guilt and feel you have to do everything for everybody. You do have time to relax but losing the guilt and anxiety and saying no occasionally might mean that you are less stressed.

Mostly b) – You are busy because you pack so much into your time that there's no chance for you to relish the good times fully. Think quality not quantity.

Mostly c) – You are busy and that's beginning to take over your life. There's not enough time to hang out with friends, and possibly family. And when you are there you're often stressed. Time to take a long hard look at how you can find more time to kick back and enjoy life.

BODY

Pump some iron

Lifting weights or strength training is the single most proactive thing you can do to ensure you stay physically active right into old age.

As you grow older, your metabolic rate decreases so that, starting around the age of 40, you can lose up to third of a pound of muscle every year. Since muscle burns off calories even when you're not using them, it means that you are likely to gain weight as muscle melts away into fat.

Remember, it's never too late to start

However, there is hope. You can either cut your calorie intake significantly or you can boost your metabolic rate. You do that by building lean muscle tissue by regular strength training. Do it regularly and you could burn an extra 300 calories a day.

But staving off weight gain is only part of the good news. According to a study of 40 postmenopausal women, after a year of strength training twice a week for 30 minutes their bodies had become as much as 15 to 20 years younger. All the participants gained bone instead of losing it as women usually do at that age, and they'd also developed muscle strength. Strong supportive muscles and a robust skeleton mean more than good posture – they make everyday movement easier and more efficient.

Remember, it's never too late to start. People between the ages of 60 and 80 increased their muscle strength by about 50% in just eight weeks of strength training. In a study of nursing home patients whose average age was 88, the group reduced body fat, increased muscle mass and saw major increases in flexibility, mobility and endurance as well as a decrease in the number of falls. In fact, the nursing home that took part in the study had to close a wing because so many residents became well enough to leave.

The anti-ageing, weight-reducing, metabolism-boosting, bone-building workout

Aim to do this at least once a week. If you have time, do it two or three times, but be sure to leave a day's rest between sessions to allow your muscles to recover. Mostly you'll be using your body as a weight. Warm up first with five minutes of marching on the spot and do some stretches at the end. In each case, do each exercise slowly and do as many repetitions as you can until you can't do any more (what's known as muscle failure). This might be 5, 10 or 20 times depending on your fitness level.

Squats with side lift

Stand with your feet slightly more than hip width apart. Lower your bottom as if you are about to sit down, hold for one breath then push yourself back up, raising your right leg out to the side as you do. Return to the start position, repeating the exercise and this time raising the left leg.

Leg lunges

Stand with your feet slightly more than hip width apart. Take a large step backwards with your right leg, placing the ball of your right foot on the floor. Slowly lower your right knee to the floor, bending your left leg as you do so. Go as low as you can before pushing off your right foot and returning to the start position. Repeat, stepping back with your left leg.

Press ups

Start on your hands and knees with your hands facing forward and in line with your shoulders, at a distance away from your body that equals approximately half your body width. Your knees should be behind your body and your back should be straight. Push down, taking the weight on your arms, until you almost reach the floor. Then push back up to the start position. Keep you abdominal muscles held tightly the whole time.

Front raises

You'll need a pair of dumb-bells for this exercise or two bottles of water. Stand with your legs slightly more than hip width apart, with your knees 'soft' (i.e. not locked). Hold your weights or water bottles by the sides of your body, palms facing downwards. Slowly raise your arms in front of your body, keeping them straight, until they are at chest height. Return to the start position and repeat.

Q and A:
All in your mind?

Q. I've heard that optimists live longer than pessimists. I'm naturally gloomy. What can I do?

A. According to psychologists, optimistic people tend to interpret their troubles as transient, controllable and specific to one situation. Pessimistic people on the other hand, believe that their troubles last forever, undermine everything they do and are completely uncontrollable. If you really are naturally gloomy – and statistics show that the number of people taking antidepressants has trebled in the past decade – psychologists believe you can actually learn to be optimistic. There's a well-documented method for building optimism that consists of recognising and disputing pessimistic thoughts. The key to disputing your own pessimistic thoughts is to first recognise them, then treat them as if they were uttered by someone else, a rival whose mission in life was to make you miserable.

Q. I am permanently exhausted but my doctor can't find anything wrong?

A. You may have Tired All The Time Syndrome (TATT). Sufferers can usually see clearly how their lifestyle isn't helping their tiredness. They just can't see how to stop it. They might be shift workers, working parents, or prone to depression. In 20–30% of sufferers there is no discernible physical problem, and in up to 50% of cases there is a psychological component. Which isn't to say that it's all in your head, but techniques such as those above where you change your thoughts may help you. The other healer is time. In one study, exhaustion did lift for the majority of the volunteers who described themselves as chronically tired. Those who recovered were markedly more likely to feel that they were generally healthy. The researchers concluded that looking after your emotional well-being and improving your general health (so you perceived yourself as a healthy person) were the best indicators that you'd make a recovery.

Q. I can't get out of bed and have had to be signed off work. Might I have ME?

A. ME or Chronic Fatigue Syndrome is a complex condition. The disease often appears to be triggered by viral illness, but often it isn't, and often although there is a viral infection, there is frequently the complication of difficult emotional circumstances. Is it a combination of both that accounts for the onset of symptoms? There are strong parallels with burnout – living a life that you've outgrown but driving yourself to succeed at it for whatever reason.

Taking extreme care of yourself physically is vital. But looking at emotional issues, too, via psychotherapy should help.

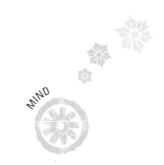

Forgive, forget, feel great

Dwelling on the past can leach away our joy in our present life, bring us down and eventually affect our health. One sure way to let go of the past is to learn to forgive. But forgiveness is not just about forgiving others. Forgiveness is also about forgiving yourself.

Things are going to happen to us that we don't like, are unfair or just plain nasty. When you forgive you make the choice to feel better about yourself and the things that have happened to you.

At the end of the day forgiveness frees up your energy

It's so easy to not want to move on but instead to wallow in self-pity. We've all been there. But if we want to lead happy lives, eventually we need to pick ourselves up because holding on to any negative feelings about another person eventually hurts us more than it could ever hurt them.

What to give up for change

Negative feelings about past events and people wastes valuable energy that you could be directing towards creating your own life and achieving your future goals. This is energy you are stealing from yourself. If the word 'forgiveness' doesn't work for you, think of it as 'moving on'. You know it's time to forgive when:

- You're harbouring resentment and bad feelings.
- You find yourself blaming others.
- You're caught up in a cycle of negative self-talk.
- You feel tired and drained.
- You're still attached to events and people from your past.
- You're working hard and not getting what you want.

At the end of the day forgiveness frees up your energy. You need this energy to get to work on your life.

Why not make a list of the benefits of holding on and the benefits of letting go. Working out what payback you are getting from not forgiving can be deeply illuminating. Focusing on the benefits of forgiving can make it seem very attractive. For example, if you have been dumped by a lover and are broken-hearted, your payback may be feeling like the virtuous martyr in front of your friends and garnering a lot of sympathy. On the other hand, if you could forgive and move on, imagine how great it would be not to care about your ex-lover any more. Think of the freedom of not caring what he was up to, who he was with. Imagine being immune to him. No matter how good it feels to be angry and bitter, not caring about him would feel infinitely better.

The Hawaiian forgiveness ritual *Ho'oponopono* is easy to do. Each morning bring to mind the person you wish to forgive. Close your eyes, take a few deep breaths and repeat the following words several times: 'I am sorry I hurt or offended you. I love you. Please forgive me.'

Yes, when you're really angry with someone, or feeling very hurt, this seems impossible and blatantly untrue. But try it and you'll find that very quickly it becomes easier. Keep repeating over weeks until it eventually feels true. And your anger and resentment will have melted away.

Forgiveness is not about forgetting or letting people off the hook. In fact, the intention of forgiveness is the opposite, to let yourself off the hook. What if you could free yourself from the emotional or psychological attachment? Wouldn't that be liberating? When you forgive, you release the person from your emotional energy. Otherwise you'll be stuck with them for years to come.

Self-forgiveness

At the end of the day the most important person you'll need to forgive is yourself. Think about how many times throughout your day you beat up on yourself with your negative thoughts and beliefs. For the next ten minutes just close your eyes and bring to mind three things you would like to forgive yourself for. Hold these in your thoughts as you repeat them to yourself several times over. Then direct the above exercise on yourself. After ten minutes open your eyes and sit quietly for a few moments before you get on with your day.

Another way of forgiving yourself is to develop a mantra that affirms your self-worth: for instance, 'I am worthy and loveable just as I am'. Write the sentence 21 times in your notebook every day. In no, time it will become true.

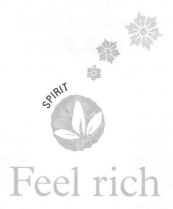

Feel rich

True wealth, both in terms of personal and financial wealth, comes from valuing who you are rather than how much you have deposited in the bank. All the money in the world won't buy you happiness.

Do you remember all those lottery winners who won millions and then lost it all? All the money in the world couldn't make them rich. What if you could work out what you were worth that wasn't based on your financial net worth but was based on your life net worth?

This exercise comes from a book called *Money Magic*, written by Deborah L. Price.

In your notebook answer the following questions:

How old are you?

How many life hours have you spent? That's your age (I'm 46) times 365 (days in the year) times 24 (hours in the day). For example, I have spent 402,960 life hours. It certainly puts a different perspective on things when you look at your life in the context of the number of hours you've lived.

How have you spent your time?

Your answer to this question can include a list of all the things you've done in your lifetime that make you feel good about who you are and the things you have done that have been meaningful to you. This is not about the things you have. Next, make a list of all the things you would still like to do that would continue to give you great fulfilment and satisfaction.

Finally, how many days are you currently spending towards meeting these personal goals?

Once you feel you have a near enough complete list, spend several minutes really taking in what you've written. How do you feel about your list? How does it feel when you look at the number of hours of your life that you've already spent? Does it make you more discerning now about how you will spend your time and money in the future? Are you really getting to live the life you want or is the way you're spending your time actually robbing you of this?

Your self-worth cannot be measured by your net worth

This exercise stretches you to consider and appreciate your worth beyond the trappings of your financial identity. You can be on the brink of bankruptcy and feel hope when you see how you have spent your time. Conversely, you can be wealthy but realise that you aren't spending your time in a way that is leading you towards your goals.

Learn to value the time that's been spent and the time left to you. With this exercise you consciously decide how you will spend it.

Whatever you have gone through, you still have your whole life ahead of you. What really matters is how you see yourself beyond what you earn. Hold on to the thought that your self-worth cannot be measured by your net worth. This recognition actually can result in more money flowing to you. And as Marlene Dietrich said: 'There's a difference between earning a great deal of money and being rich'.

Feel rich instantly

Start a gratitude journal. Every day, write down three things that you appreciate and value from your day. Include the small incidents in your day, such as someone offering you a seat on a packed commuter train, or the bus driver who let you out on a very busy junction. Go from the least obvious to the most obvious. Soon you will reach the stage where you feel immensely grateful and successful for simply waking up in your own bed.

Four

Optimum health

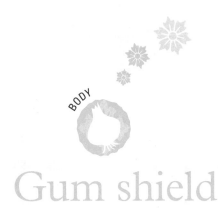

BODY

Gum shield

Protecting your mouth against gum disease is just about the simplest life-saving strategy you can undertake. It costs virtually nothing and takes around two minutes a day.

How often do you floss your teeth? It's one of those things that we all intend to do more often than we actually do. Here's a hint: if you've had a packet of floss for more than a month, you're not flossing enough. But there's compelling evidence that flossing should be as much second nature as brushing our teeth. It will help you live longer. In fact, flossing your teeth every day is such a powerful health protector it can take almost six and a half years off your real age, according to US anti-ageing guru Dr Michael Roizen.

Flossing is vital as it's the most effective way of staving off gum disease. And gum disease, left untreated, can lead to inflammation of the arteries, a major precursor to heart disease.

Gum disease starts when plaque, which is a mix of bacteria, saliva and food debris is left for long periods on the gum surface. If it is undisturbed for around a day, the bacteria reproduce and start to become toxic, infecting the gums. It's unfair, but women are more prone than men to gum disease because of hormonal changes that weaken the body's ability to fight the effect of bacteria on the gums. These bacteria can be sucked into the lungs during breathing, where they cross into the bloodstream and are carried to various parts of the body. This triggers an immune response which causes inflammation throughout the body – including the arteries.

In its first stage, gum disease is known as gingivitis. The main symptom is gums which bleed easily – you may notice blood on your toothbrush or when you rinse your mouth. Another major sign is bad breath that disappears when you brush your teeth, only to return soon afterwards. If you see blood you need to floss more often and see a dentist or hygienist for advice. Most gingivitis clears within two to three weeks with rigorous attention to oral hygiene.

Gingivitis is easily treated with good oral hygiene; if ignored, it can lead to periodontal disease where the gums recede and bacteria attack the bone supporting the teeth. Unless it's treated with antibiotics, the teeth may eventually fall out. But this is only one reason to take periodontitis very seriously. It's linked with an increased risk of stroke, and scientists have found that bacteria which grow in the mouth can be drawn into the lungs to cause respiratory diseases such as pneumonia. Severe periodontal disease can also include blood sugar levels. In addition, gum disease is the number one cause of tooth loss for older people.

How to prevent gum disease

1   *Use an electric toothbrush twice a day.* Electric toothbrushes are 25% more effective than conventional brushes at removing plaque. There's also a correct

technique to brushing – hold the brush at a 45 degree angle to the gumline and move the brush back and forth in short strokes. Change your toothbrush or brush head every two to three months.

2   *Floss once a day.* When we brush we tend to reach only two surfaces of the tooth – the front and back. Bacteria are left to multiply on the surfaces between them. But 90% of gum disease is caused by the bacteria left undisturbed between the teeth. It's vital to floss at least once a day so the bacteria are dislodged and don't reach the toxic stage. If you find you're too tired to do it last thing at night and don't have time in the morning, do it while you're watching TV or sitting in traffic. (Store it next to your remote or in the glove compartment.)

3   *Use mouthwash twice a day.* Antibacterial mouth rinses dislodge bacteria left behind by brushing. But don't use one which contains alcohol, as it will dry out the mouth and encourage the bacteria to breed further.

4   *See a dental hygienist regularly.* You should see a dental hygienist every six months or more often if you are diagnosed with gum disease. A hygienist can painlessly remove all the plaque that's accumulated around the gums and under the gumline.

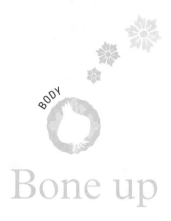

BODY

Bone up

Nothing speaks of youth like a strong, supple spine. Building strong bones will keep you looking years younger for much longer and safeguard your health when you actually are old.

Our bones do naturally become weaker with age, but they should remain strong enough to support us as long as we're alive. However, in some people the skeleton starts crumbling at a faster than normal rate, leading to osteoporosis. It affects one third of all women.

The bones are made of a thick outer shell and strong inner mesh filled with collagen (protein), calcium salts and other minerals. The inside looks like honeycomb with blood vessels and bone marrow in the spaces between bone. Osteoporosis occurs when the holes between the honeycomb become bigger, making it fragile and liable to break easily. Osteoporosis usually affects the whole skeleton but it most commonly causes fractures in the wrist, spine and hip. But the good news is that bone is alive and constantly changing. Old, worn out bone is broken down and replaced by bone-building cells called osteoblasts. This process of renewal is called bone turnover. And there's much you can do to increase your bone turnover and improve your bone strength – whatever your age.

Eating a bone-friendly diet is your first step. You probably already know that calcium is essential. You need around 700–1000mg a day, which could get from say, a half pint of semi-skimmed milk, a low-fat yogurt, and a pot of low-fat cottage cheese. As a general rule, include dairy products at two to three meals, and drink milk in tea and coffee. Other good sources are leafy green vegetables, baked beans, dried fruit, almonds and oily fish such as sardines, pilchards or anchovies where you eat the bones. You can also get a little from tap water if you live in a hard water area.

To be on the safe side, it's best to take a calcium supplement. Look for one that contains vitamin D which helps the body absorb calcium. There is also research to show that the omega-3 fish oils work in tandem with calcium, so look for supplements that combine these nutrients.

But note that if you are taking a fish *liver* oil (such as cod liver oil), think of switching to a fish oil. If you are taking a fish liver oil plus a multivitamin you may be taking in quite high levels of vitamin A – too much puts you at risk of broken bones. You shouldn't be getting more than 1500mg of vitamin A per day.

A very important strategy is to exercise. Weight bearing exercise (where you are subject to gravity so that your body acts as a weight) is what's needed (so swimming and cycling don't count). Putting repetitive stress on the bones stimulates new bone formation. Walking, jogging, aerobics, dancing or yoga all help.

More care needed?

A bone scan measures the density of your bones and compares this to a normal range so it can tell you if you look like being the one woman in three likely to succumb to bone disease. See your doctor to discuss your options if:

- You've broken a bone after a minor fall.
- You've been through a premature menopause (before 45).
- You've had a hysterectomy.
- You've missed periods for more than six months (not due to pregnancy).
- You've been on corticosteroid tablets for long periods for conditions such as arthritis or asthma.
- You've got a family history of osteoporosis.

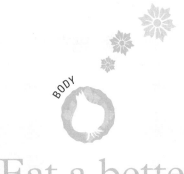

Eat a better breakfast

If you eat breakfast you are 50% less likely to have blood-sugar problems and you reduce your chances of being overweight by one third. All this plus more energy and mental focus. So how do you maximise the potential of this one meal to improve your health?

The best fuel combination is a carbohydrate and protein breakfast. Carbohydrate releases energy quickly (it gives you the boost to run for the bus), but protein releases energy for longer (it will help you clinch the deal during that tricky pre-lunch conference call). If you eat carbs alone in the morning or nothing at all, your body may well crave more carbs at 11 a.m. – hence the doughnut run that wreaks such damage to your figure and your idea of yourself as a person with self-control. So remember: carbs good; a bit of protein essential. Here are some ideas.

OK breakfast

Bowl of non-sugary cereal (Shreddies, All-Bran) with semi-skimmed or skimmed milk. Piece of fruit or good quality juice.

How to make it better

The milk provides some protein, but not much. Nibble on a little hard cheese or cottage cheese, or have a slice of cheese on wholemeal toast to get some protein in there.

Better breakfast

Porridge with plain yogurt and a handful of seeds and dried fruit and/or a teaspoon of honey to sweeten.

How to make it better

You may find that the yogurt does enough to fill you up, but probably not always. Again, try cheese, or a handful of nuts on top of the porridge.

Best breakfast

- Scrambled eggs on wholegrain toast.
- Mackerel or kippers with wholegrain toast.
- Smoked salmon and cream cheese on wholegrain toast or bagel.
- Omelette with cheese, tomato and mushrooms.

How to make it better

Add a piece of fruit and you're set to go.

Breakfast is the forgotten meal, when actually it should be the focus of our food intake. It would be better for you to eat dinner as your first meal of the day, but realistically, most of us can't or wouldn't want to eat that much first thing.

Here are two liquid breakfasts for those who really hate the idea of eating in the morning. These are excellent sources of all the nutrients you need and should keep you full until lunch.

- *Chicken soup*: Why not? Chicken soup is a marvellous breakfast on a cold morning, or any morning, and is how the Chinese start off the day. You can make it ahead of time and heat it up in seconds. Treat yourself to a special bowl, perhaps Chinese in design, and sip your soup in a Zen like way. Sauté leeks and onions together in a little olive oil then add a minced garlic clove and cook until they are transparent. Add potatoes, carrots, chicken stock, a handful of shredded chicken. Throw in a pinch of nutmeg, grated ginger or horseradish if you like. After you've brought to the boil, leave to simmer for 15 minutes or so until the hard vegetables are cooked and just before serving, toss in some pak choi, spinach, curly kale or watercress – any greens. You can liquidise or keep it chunky. Add some noodles, too, for the authentic Chinese experience.

- *A smoothie*: Mix half a pint of ice-cold, semi-skimmed or soya milk with a banana, a pinch of cinnamon and two teaspoons of fish or flaxseed oil. Throw in a handful of soft fruits such as raspberries, blueberries or strawberries. (Out of season, you can buy frozen packets of these in supermarkets.) Sip with a handful of nuts.

Kate Winslet's
health plan

Kate Winslet has confessed to never feeling completely OK in her own skin because of weight issues when she was younger. Her health plan is based on staying slim and fit without taking it to extremes.

She finds ways to motivate herself

She hates workouts, so runs on a treadmill in front of the TV five to seven times a week. 'Everyone can commit to 20 minutes of working out especially if there's a glass of Chardonnay afterwards,' she says.

She doesn't eat what doesn't suit her

She has cut out bread from her diet as she thinks it disagrees with her. She has also cut right down on other processed foods.

She thinks positively

She works on her self-esteem and doesn't put her body down in case her young daughter picks up any negative self-image habits from her. 'I work on loving my backside,' she says.

BODY

Happy holidays

If you've ever spent your holidays being either stressed or ill, then it's time to take steps to use them to promote health benefits.

'Leisure sickness', a.k.a. 'stop and collapse' syndrome, is a fact of modern life. The very times that we put aside to relax and recuperate are wasted being sick. A study of nearly 2000 people discovered that a small but significant number regularly got ill at the weekend or on holidays. The main symptoms are headaches, migraine, fatigue, muscular pains, nausea, colds and flu.

Those who get it share certain characteristics: a high workload, perfectionism, eagerness to achieve, an overdeveloped sense of responsibility to their work – all of these make it difficult to switch off.

The most obvious way of ending the syndrome is of course to give up the above habits and thus reduce stress. But given that might not be an option immediately, there are two ways to tackle this problem.

1   Support your immune system. At a very bare minimum, eat five portions of fruit and veg a day and take good quality multivitamin and mineral supplements. If you drink alcohol every day or are a smoker, you need vitamin C, too.
2   Plan for holidays well in advance. Start packing three weeks in advance and gathering everything you need.

Sort a work schedule two weeks in advance, planning what tasks you need to commit and when you're going to complete them (preferably one day before your last day).

Christmas is a special holiday, one that can also lead to 'crash and burn' even if there's no passport involved. Two-thirds of women report feeling stressed and worn out after the Christmas holidays.

The above advice still holds, of course. Get into peak condition and plan, plan, plan. Start Christmas shopping and card writing in November and you'll find that there's less chance of keeling over with stress.

In addition there are two strategies that really help reduce stress:

1   The one-day shopping blitz. Allow yourself just one day to buy presents. Limit yourself to one store. Research shows that if we limit choice we make decisions faster and we're happier with those decisions. If you do your shopping on the internet, adopt the same policy.

Otherwise you'll spend days browsing rather than deciding. A time limit focuses the brain.

2   The cut-off point. Decide on an hour, probably sometime on Christmas Eve, when you stop. Whatever isn't done by that time doesn't get done – and that is a powerful motivation to serenely reach your goal. At the cut-off point, sit down, relax and begin to enjoy your Christmas.

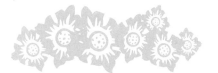

Feel good now: *Drinking a glass of red wine a day keeps you healthier than teetotallers. But obviously, much more than this and you cancel out the good effects.*

What to eat every day

This isn't a comprehensive list of everything you should eat in a day, but stick it on your fridge and aim to include this list each day, and you'll see significant improvements in your health and well-being. These are the basics for keeping you calm and energetic.

Every day eat…

- One orange – for vitamin C (or another helping of vitamin C food).
- One helping of oats, fish, meat or eggs (for vitamin B, necessary for beating stress).
- One helping of broccoli or one helping of carrots (brilliant for antioxidants).
- Two to three servings of reduced fat dairy which is rich in natural opiates called casmorphins, which keep you calm and energetic.

Guidelines

- *Lunch*. One small serving of good-quality carbohydrate. Too much and you'll feel dozy but one slice of wholegrain bread or a fist-sized portion of wholegrain pasta or rice will release the feelgood hormone serotonin.
- *Dinner*. One small portion of good quality protein.

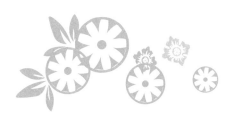

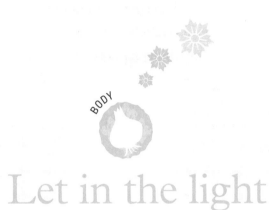

Let in the light

Most of us have heard of SAD – Seasonal Affective Disorder – but are less aware that there are millions of people affected by the 'sub-syndrome'.

You may not have SAD, but if you feel downhearted and/or exhausted all winter you could be one of them.

Before electricity, everything changed for our ancestors during the winter months. Lack of daylight affected every part of their lives. Now we can work and play around the clock: the lack of light need never impinge upon our lifestyle. But that doesn't mean that lack of daylight doesn't have a profound effect on us. Normal electric lights can't replace daylight as far as our bodies are concerned.

- Do you dread the winter months?
- Do you tend to put on weight in winter?
- Do you find it near impossible to get out of bed in the morning when it's dark outside?
- Do you find you are more paranoid or self-doubting in winter?

Answer yes to two or more and lack of light could be affecting you. The further north you live, the more likely you are to be affected by the lack of light.

What can you do?

Step 1   Get outside for half an hour a day during the winter months. Make it a habit to go for a walk at lunchtime but since sunlight is so precious in the UK during winter, if at all possible, think about dropping everything, making your excuses and getting outside as soon as the sun comes out whatever the time of day.

Step 2   If you still feel blue, St John's Wort has been proven to help with the symptoms of SAD. It is not suitable for those on some other medications including the Pill and some heart drugs. It is also helpful in combating overeating linked with mild depression.

Step 3   Invest in a light box which supplies doses of strong white light as you work or sit in your home. Light therapy is more effective than Prozac in treating SAD: 95% of its users reported it improved their condition, and 85% see an improvement after three to four days of around two hours treatment. You can buy one via the internet or at a chemist or health food shop.

A one-minute answer to mid-afternoon slump

Practically, every medical system in the world (with the exception of our own) believes that energy flows around the body in channels. Suspend disbelief!

Lack of energy is attributed to a block somewhere in this energy flow. Release the block and you get increased energy. You can do this by applying needles, fingers or elbows to specific acupuncture points around the body. Evidence shows that acupressure works for helping with post-operative nausea and lower back pain, and although there is no such research into this facial massage, mastering gives you a terrific tool to relieve tiredness and mental exhaustion anytime you need it. It's specially useful when you spend a lot of time at your desk.

Shiatsu facial massage for instant energy boost

- Lean your elbows on a table and let your face drop into your hands with your palms cupped over your eyes. Look into the darkness formed by your hands. Stay there for as long as you feel comfortable or until your colleagues start to get worried.

- Place your thumbs on the inner end of each eyebrow and use your index fingers to work out along the upper edge of the eyebrow, applying pressure at regular intervals. When your index fingers reach the outer edge of your eyebrow, release all pressure.

- Return index finger to the inner end of each brow and work thumbs along to the lower end of the brows in similar fashion. Release as before.

- Place thumbs under ear lobes and apply pressure. At the same time, use the index fingers to apply pressure on points on a line from the bridge of the nose under your eyes, along the ridge formed by your eye sockets.

- Touch fingertips to fingertips along an imaginary line running up the middle of your forehead from your nose to your hairline (no pressure is necessary). Use thumbs to apply pressure to points fanning out from the outer edge of the eyebrows to hairline. Repeat four times. (Feel for tender points and massage them.)

- Use thumbs to apply gentle pressure in the eye sockets under the inner end of the eyebrow where you feel the ridge of the eye socket. (This is a very delicate spot so go gently.)

- Use one index finger to work up that imaginary line in your mid-forehead from the nose to your hairline.

- Now drop your head forward and, lifting your arms, work your thumbs from your spine outwards along the ridge of your skull from the spine out to the point just under your ear lobes. Do this four times.

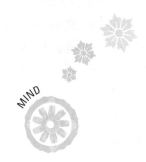

Change your attitude, stay young

We can learn a lot about longevity from Oscar winners. It seems that the more successful you are, the longer you live. But it depends on your definition of success.

On average, Oscar winners live four years longer than non-Oscar winning actors, and actors winning many Academy Awards live an average of six years longer.

But you don't have to be rich and a celebrity. What makes a difference to your health is being socially successful. Your position in the social hierarchy is what matters. If you want to live a long life, you need to scramble to the top of your particular social pile. How much money you have is unimportant – provided you feel you have more than those around you. Being seen as a success and held in esteem by your peer group has a powerful effect on the immune system. It's also boosted by feeling that you're in control of your life. Lack of control leads to high stress levels and that leads to increased rates of heart disease, stroke and even cancer.

What aspects of your job are beyond your control? Is there anything you can do to change the situation? If not, can you change how you react to the situation? What aspect of your job empowers you? Can you do more of it?

If there's not much you can do about your job, concentrate on being popular instead. It's thought that being held in high esteem by your close friends and family, and having plenty of opportunities to get out and meet people, can counteract the negative, ageing effects of a poor job.

A youthful mental image of yourself is vital if you want to stave off ageing

It's up to you how you define success. It could mean turning down a well-paid job to do something you find more fulfilling. It could be feeling fitter, stronger and more vital with every year. Or it could be as simple as being honest and authentic in your dealings with other people at all times. Take a few minutes to write down what success means to you and write down a short description. It's always easier to work towards a goal that's clearly defined.

Mind games

There are other ways of changing your attitude that can help you stay young in mind and body. Our mind and body are inextricably lined. Each cell in your body communicates with all the other cells to enable the body to work as one unit. So changes in the brain's cellular activity caused by various emotions will have a direct impact on all the other cells in your body.

What makes for a healthy, useful mindset? It's important to ditch guilt. Research has shown that people with low levels of guilt are less likely to suffer from colds or flu. It has been discovered that guilt over enjoying things like sex or eating chocolate lowers levels of immunoglobulin A, which is associated with a strong immune system.

A youthful mental image of yourself is vital if you want to stave off ageing. Your mind is like a heat-seeking missile – it moves towards the goals you create, be they positive or negative. So think of yourself as a youthful, energetic person and you'll start to act like one. Think 'I want to be someone who looks ten years younger and has enormous amounts of energy and zest for life.' Then ask yourself, what actions would this person take? What would they eat? How would they deal with stress? How would they start each day?

It takes about three weeks for a repetitive action to form new pathways in the brain and become a habit. So try making one change at a time and sticking at it for three weeks before tackling another. Start with something small such as flossing your teeth or eating two extra pieces of fruit a day.

Let down your defences

Are you aware of the patterns of defensive behaviour that you've cultivated over time that act as a form of protection against people, events or experiences that have caused you pain? Recognising and dealing with them can eliminate stress and increase happiness.

We recognise when friends and family are 'becoming defensive' but we're not so great at recognising it in ourselves. All of us have erected defences early on in childhood as a way of protecting ourselves from painful or difficult emotions and traumas. Your memories of your personal traumas and painful emotions get stored in a part of the brain called the amygdala, which also stores all your reactions to those experiences – whether you lashed out, froze, acted out in rage or became a victim. Some of these reactions become our preferred method of dealing with pain – our defence mechanisms. These serve you well and help you journey from childhood to adulthood.

But you often outgrow the psychological and emotional responses and behaviours. They have helped you so far but now you need different, better tools to deal with life's problems.

Your first step is to get clear on what your defence mechanisms are.

- Think of three specific challenges you've dealt with.
- What behaviours or patterns did you adopt to cope with each challenge?

- On a scale of 0–10, with 10 meaning the defence still works well (helps you in life) and 0 meaning the defence isn't working well at all (it makes you unhappy or limits your life), rate the defence in its current working order today.

Answering these questions requires self-honesty. It may mean getting in touch with sadness or resentment. It may mean you have to remember times when you wished you'd acted differently.

It may well mean you stepping out of your comfort zone.

For instance, if you handle criticism by withdrawing into yourself and putting up barriers, you may discover that this defence mechanism, although keeping you safe from being hurt, means that you don't have a wide circle of friends. You may even dread making social contact and be perceived as a loner by those around you. It has become limiting.

Next step would be replacing the old defence mechanism with a new strategy that serves you better. For instance, if the above example was your problem, you could perhaps spend a few minutes several times a day, visualising yourself inviting colleagues out for a sandwich at lunchtime, calling friends who haven't been in your life for a while or in other ways including yourself in social events. And imagine these going incredibly well. This will change your attitudes towards others and soon, what seemed daunting, will have become an active pleasure.

The next time you feel a familiar pattern kicking in, practise changing your response to the pattern. So let's say, for example, your normal pattern is to eat whenever you feel threatened or anxious. The feelings of anxiety and being threatened become your triggers. You defend yourself from the anxious emotions or the discomfort of feeling threatened by reaching for food. To break the pattern, interrupt the behaviour by inserting a substitute response. So instead of going straight downstairs to the kitchen, take a detour and head for your notebook and write for ten minutes about the feelings and emotions that have been stirred up inside you.

For more support have a read of *The Writing Diet* by Julia Cameron. Bear in mind this quote from famous psychologist and author, Dorothy Rowe: 'Defences keep us stuck in one unhappy place. It takes truth and courage to abandon them, but once we do, we discover a world of freedom and wonderful possibilities.'

Index